What early readers & medical professionals are saying:

» "From one of the bariatric community's thought leaders comes a must read guide for any patient, primary care physician or bariatric surgeon considering bariatric surgery as a treatment for morbid obesity. Dr. Sasse takes us through a journey of hope, without sugar-coating the risk involved in this life changing operation and outlines the key steps to becoming a healthier and happy person through successful preoperative and postoperative treatment plans. Bariatric surgery has been called the most effective tool in the treatment of morbid obesity. This book is the operational manual of that tool."

— Dr. Kevin Huffman, Medical Director of the American Bariatric Centers, President American Bariatric Consultants

» "Dr. Sasse presents an inspiring and thought provoking approach to weight loss. He takes note of what works and what doesn't. He includes important lessons on how to succeed in the field of weight loss. His expertise is unquestioned, yet his advice is so approachable. It is like having your own personal guide helping you with one of the most challenging endeavors in life: losing weight and keeping it off. This Guide is destined to become a standard reference for both potential patients and health care providers involved in the field of weight loss medicine and surgery."

— Laurie McGinley, MS, CNS-BC, APN, CBN--- President, National Association of Bariatric Nurses (NABN)

» "This is an amazing book for the patient or professional who wants to learn about weight loss surgery. It is the kind of book every surgeon and every surgery center should provide to prospective patients. I learned more about the subject in a couple of hours of reading this book than I'd learned in years of anecdotes about bariatric surgery."

– SCOTT BECKER, JD, CPA, HARVARD LAW SCHOOL '89, PUBLISHER BECKERS ASC REVIEW, CO CHAIR MCGUIREWOODS HEALTHCARE PRACTICE

» "What an insightful guide for patients seeking to lose weight! But this book is also a highly informative guide for Ambulatory center leaders, health care administrators and personnel who will now understand the coming tide of outpatient procedures for weight loss. "One of the best personal health books I have ever read. A unique combination of fascinating technology and powerful inspiration."

– JOHN H. GANSER, M.D., FACS

» "Dr. Kent Sasse has written the quintessential book on weight loss surgery. Informative without being overwhelming, Dr. Sasse explains the process in an explicit, concise way beneficial to both the mildly curious and those seriously considering this life-changing procedure. Having had the surgery with Dr. Sasse I can truly say that he has laid out the options with all their benefits and risks. Reading his book would give anyone the knowledge and information needed to decide on whether this innovate approach to life long health should be in their future."

– KATHY BURKE, WEIGHT LOSS SURGERY PATIENT

» "Dr. Sasse brings compassion and an insightful look into the window of surgical weight loss…. with the most up to date information in the industry. Dr. Sasse has performed over 2000 surgeries and has made weight management his life's passion only speaks to his integrity. If you read only one book on weight loss surgery this is it…"

– CHEF DAVE FOUTS, THE WORLD'S FIRST BARIATRIC CHEF,
AUTHOR, 90 WAYS TO DITCH YOUR DIET

» "It took 50 years, but Dr. Sasse has re-defined the weight loss standard. He is known for his professionalism and is loved by his patients. His book is the culmination of his work to date in this very important field. A must read for anyone considering their options for weight loss surgery."

– THOMAS MALLON, CEO, REGENT SURGICAL HEALTH,
CHICAGO, ILLINOIS

» "Not only is his book a help guide and knowledge manual, but it also inspires the reader to see how they CAN DO IT and how they WILL SUCCEED! I will use it to hand out to my Life Coaching clients who are considering both surgical and non-surgical weight loss."

– RICHARD CUNNINGHAM, PROFESSIONAL LIFE COACH

» "An extremely comprehensive look into the most powerful tool for effective long-term weight loss. Dr. Sasse goes far beyond procedural details and provides an all-encompassing look into bariatric weight loss surgery. Written by one of the foremost experts in the medical weight loss field, Outpatient Weight Loss Surgery is an absolutely essential guide for anyone considering weight loss surgery."

– STEPHEN B. MAYVILLE, PH.D., B.C.B.A.
LICENSED CLINICAL PSYCHOLOGIST
DIRECTOR OF PSYCHOLOGICAL SERVICES,
THE INTERNATIONAL METABOLIC INSTITUTE

» "Full of practical wisdom and insight, Dr. Sasse's Guide to Outpatient Weight Loss Surgery provides real-life examples and testimonials plus a careful, experienced surgeon's advice about how to achieve the best results. This book will help many people change their lives for the better."

– COLLEEN COOK, PRESIDENT
BARIATRIC SUPPORT CENTERS INTERNATIONAL,
AUTHOR, THE SUCCESS HABITS OF WEIGHT LOSS SURGERY PATIENTS

» "Dr. Sasse has managed to pull together what is surely to become an industry standard. Coupling clear, concise and easy to understand information with real life examples from his own practice, Dr. Sasse pulls together both the clinical and the practical in a style sure to be a hit with patients."

– REGI SCHINDLER, PRESIDENT & CEO, BLIS, INC

Outpatient Weight-Loss Surgery

Safe and Successful Weight Loss With Modern Bariatric Surgery

A Sasse Guide

Kent Sasse, M.D., MPH, FACS

360 Publishing

Reno, Nevada

A portion of the proceeds from this book go to support the Obesity Prevention Foundation.

Edited by Cindie Geddes, Flying Hand Services and Jennifer Baumer.
Inside pages designed by Jessie Gardner, JG Designers, Inc.
Cover designed by Anita Jones, Another Jones Graphics.

The author is grateful for permission to include the following previously copyrighted materials and images:
Ethicon EndoSurgery, Allergan Corporation, Covidian and EndoGastric Solutions

Publisher's Cataloging-In-Publication Data
(Prepared by The Donohue Group, Inc.)

Sasse, Kent.
  Outpatient weight-loss surgery : safe and successful weight loss with modern bariatric surgery / Kent Sasse.

    p. : ill. ; cm. -- (Sasse guide)

  Includes bibliographical references and index.
  ISBN: 978-1-934727-00-3

1. Obesity--Surgery--Popular works. 2. Gastric bypass--Popular works. 3. Weight loss--Popular works. I. Title.

RD605 .S27 2009
617.4/3

Acknowledgements

I AM DEEPLY INDEBTED to so many people who have helped to make this book possible and who have helped in its research and writing. First and foremost, I would like to thank my patients, who perform the daily miracles of fighting this disease of obesity, and who challenge me and my colleagues to be better caregivers and better people.

I am indebted to so many people at the International Metabolic Institute and Western Bariatric Institute for their hard work and dedication to our patients and to the work of combating this disease. To Tiffany Rice, Sarai Swanson, Roberta Brown, Kimberly Brown, Donna Wainscoat, Jennifer Padgett, Trees Lonis-Muller, Billie Keuper, Patrick Allen, Gayleen Gott-Anderson, Jenna Beh, Curtis Smith, Darolyn Skelton, Laramie Lathrop, Laurie McGinley, Marte Lyson, Mason Hermosillo, Nicole Walker, Vicki Bovee, Dr. Kozar, Dr. Ganser, Dr. Watson, Cindi Lee, Gregory Bowman, Mark Conte, Tracy Visher, Natasha Mulqueen, Dr. Pamela Corson, Doina Kulick, Dr. Michael Bloch, Dr. Kristina Hansen, Stephen Mayville, PhD, Brie Moore, PhD, Dennis Fitzpatrick, Robin Marquez, RN, Anne Lazarus,

Jennifer Baumer, Cindie Geddes, Jessie Gardner and Anita Jones have done an amazing job with editing and designing this book. Dionne Lim has been an outstanding research assistant and investigator of facts. I would also like to thank Craig Belis and Jason Green, Joanne McCall and Sharon Castlen for their hard work, patience, dedication, and sense of humor.

And special thanks to Norma Seed, Karen Mitchell, Margi Houk, Richard Cunningham, Terry Beauchamp, Carol Bradley, Karen Fisher, Richard Cunningham, Eleanor Houk, Beth Devine, Debby Howard, Jonda Jones, Mike Darragh, Nancy Guthery, Sherrill Sundell, Anita Acosta, Karen Mitchell, Kathy Burke, Mary Francis, Debby Howard, and Jonda Jones.

Dedication

To my children, Alexandra and Olivia,
who provide life's inspiration.

Foreword

IN RECENT YEARS, pioneering surgeons have applied sophisticated minimally-invasive surgical techniques to the practice of weight loss surgery, known as bariatric surgery. Long term studies now clearly demonstrate profound improvements in the lives of overweight people who undergo the surgery. The benefits are striking and range from markedly longer lifespan, to improvements in quality of life, to the resolution of diabetes, hypertension, sleep apnea and many other serious diseases. Today, weight gain and obesity adversely affect the lives of a billion people around the world, and solutions that are less invasive and more demonstrably effective are more available now more than ever.

From participating in the initial stages of metabolic and weight loss surgery, to witnessing the most recent innovations in technical medical gadgetry, it has been immensely gratifying to see my earliest and most optimistic vision of what this surgery could mean to so many people now become manifest. When I authored the widely cited paper, Outcomes After laparoscopic Roux-en-Y gastric bypass for morbid obesity (Annals of Surgery

232(4):515-529, October, 2000), few in the medical community or lay public understood the impact that weight loss surgery could have on an individual person's life, let alone its impact on an overweight society.

That impact is now occurring daily, as over 200,000 people undergo weight loss surgery annually in the U.S. alone. And if this book has the kind of impact I believe it will, that number is likely to rise significantly.

Over the last 40 years I have had the honor of leading the field of weight loss medicine and surgery toward real solutions that work for real people. With great effort and perseverance, and against many obstacles, devoted surgeons discovered techniques that profoundly and favorably affected the lives of overweight people, leading them to dramatically reduce their weight and live longer, healthier lives. These early interventions were invasive, open procedures with higher risks and complications than we would accept today. They led to newer and better procedures, and paved the way for the modern minimally-invasive weight loss revolution chronicled in this book.

Dr. Sasse's book, Outpatient Weight Loss Surgery, is stunning not only because the existence of such a book was unthinkable only a few years ago, but also because of the clarity and succinctness with which Dr. Sasse explores the terrain of modern weight loss surgery.

If you or someone you love is overweight or obese, then the book you are holding in your hand is nothing short of essential reading material. This is one of the first books that explains the revolution of modern, minimally invasive, highly-effective weight loss surgery and its transition to the outpatient environment. If you or someone you care about has even considered weight loss surgery, I strongly recommend that you read this book for its candid and insightful information and guidance.

What we are witnessing with the publication of this book is a sea-change in the treatment of obesity. As chronicled by Dr. Sasse, long gone are the days when a seriously overweight person had few medical professionals to whom he or she could turn. Long gone are the days when medicine offered little hope for an obese person seeking answers. Forty years ago, surgery was invasive and as yet unproven, and fad diets and dubious injections attracted customers who had few proven alternatives. What is perhaps most striking about the publication of this book is that it marks a turning point to a time in which effective proven, minimally-invasive solutions exist for long term weight loss and health improvement. As this book makes abundantly clear, that time is now.

One of the great tragedies over recent years has been that old stereotypes and the lack of fresh information have deterred many doctors from recommending weight loss surgery and have deterred countless millions of obese patients from seeking it. As numerous studies have now demonstrated, that has led to so much unnecessary suffering, disease and early mortality from obesity.

It is my hope that with the reach of this book, and the greater and more widespread understanding of the impact of obesity on a person's health, that more people who so desperately need it can avail themselves of this valuable medical treatment. Perhaps the move to less and less invasive techniques and the shift to the out-patient arena will inspire more doctors to recommend the proce-dure and more obese patients to investigate it.

Weight loss surgery is not for everyone and Dr. Sasse's sober and candid discussion of not only the benefits but also the risks and complications associated with weight loss surgery make it valuable reading for anyone considering weight loss treatments or any doctor recommending them.

– PHILLIP SCHAUER, MD
DIRECTOR, BARIATRIC SURGERY PROGRAM CLEVELAND CLINIC
PAST PRESIDENT, AMERICAN SOCIETY FOR METABOLIC AND
BARIATRIC SURGEONS

Table of Contents

About the Author

Dr. Kent C. Sasse, M.D., MPH, FACS

K ENT SASSE, MD, MPH, FACS is a nationally renowned authority on surgical weight-loss procedures and a leader in the rapidly evolving field of bariatric surgery. The distinguished recipient of several awards, including membership in the prestigious Alpha Omega Alpha Society for top medical graduates in the country, Dr. Sasse is founder and medical director of both the iMetabolic International Metabolic Institute and Western Bariatric Institute, a nationally recognized ASMBS Center of Excellence.

The recipient of a bachelor's degree in biochemistry at the University of California San Diego, where he graduated cum laude, and two master's degrees, including a master's degree in public health stemming from research related to biostatistics and bioethics, from the University of California Berkeley, Dr. Sasse completed residency training in surgery, focusing on gastrointestinal surgery and physiology, at the University of California San Francisco, as well as fellowship training at the Lahey Clinic in Boston, Massachusetts, before establishing his practice in northern Nevada.

Dedicated to the highest levels of scientific research and individualized, state-of-the-art treatment of patients, Dr. Sasse brings a wealth of experience and expertise to the rapidly evolving field of weight-loss surgery. He has written and continues to pursue several IRB-approved research protocols regarding weight loss and weight-loss surgery, and he lectures frequently on topics related to obesity and weight reduction at the University of Nevada School of Medicine. Through his nationally recognized programs, Dr. Sasse and his outstanding faculty provide patients the highest levels of compassionate medicine, scientific evidence, and personalized care in the field of weight reduction.

*Please visit **www.sasseguide.com** for more information on Dr. Sasse and his world-renowned programs and facilities.*

Introduction

FIFTEEN YEARS AGO, this book would have been highly unlikely. Because 15 years ago, it was more than unlikely – it was unthinkable – that the most effective, durable and widely popular surgical weight-loss procedures could be performed as outpatient procedures.

Technology, technique and need have combined in the last 15 years, and today we stand at a remarkable moment in time when the most successful, proven, life-prolonging weight-loss treatments have passed from unproven to the land of the tested, tried and true. Surgical weight-loss procedures were once complex and rarely performed due to the high risk and the uncertainty of the outcomes. Today technological and medical advances have made surgical weight-loss procedures more effective, less invasive, less risky, more convenient and private, and there are much shorter recovery times.

Need alone has greatly advanced the science of bariatric surgery. Unprecedented numbers of people in this country are significantly overweight and looking for ways to help themselves feel

better, look better and live longer, healthier lives. If you or someone you love is struggling to lose weight, you probably already
know the health risks associated with being overweight and the
health benefits associated with losing weight.

While it is true that today more people worldwide are overweight than have been ever before, it is also true that there are
more effective and less invasive solutions than there ever have
been before. Today, unprecedented numbers of people are choosing outpatient surgical weight-loss procedures for the convenience
and tremendous health benefits. And in the very near future, even
more people will learn about outpatient weight-loss solutions and
take advantage of them.

This book was written in order to share the revolution taking place in the field of weight-loss treatment. The evolution
of outpatient surgical weight-loss procedures and the cutting
edge technology evolving within the field of bariatric surgery is
exciting but not widely known. In this book, I'll explain rapidly
evolving state-of-the-art weight-loss treatments and touch on
advances in experimental treatments, including some that are
nonsurgical.

This book provides accurate, unbiased, up-to-date information
and demystifies the emerging technology of surgical weight-loss
procedures so you can make informed decisions on any weight-

loss solutions you may be considering. It is a both a guide to weight-loss success in the modern era of outpatient treatments and a chronicle of the weight-loss treatment revolution taking place today.

It's time to start living the life you've imagined.

– HENRY JAMES

1

The Outpatient Revolution

A S RECENTLY AS the 1980s, bariatric (or weight-loss) procedures were major, open, full-anesthetic operations performed in the clinical confines of hospital operating rooms. A large incision had to be made, which ran up the abdomen from below the bellybutton to the breastbone and cut through the major abdominal muscles, which are not forgiving of such intrusions and do not heal easily or quickly. Clearly such surgical procedures required a significant stay in the hospital, and complications occurred frequently.

If you first started hearing about bariatric surgery during the 1970s and early 80s, you probably remember it as being a frightening surgical procedure with frequent complications, such as the formation of hernias (or bulges of the muscle incisions), and problems that arose from infection, and breathing difficulties. (While any surgical procedure can impair lung function to some degree because of anesthesia, being overweight can stress the lungs even more after an operation, leading to complications such as pneumonia.) In those early days, weight-loss operations were considered less than elective, more often performed because excess weight had put the patient at risk for imminent health complications such as diabetes or heart failure.

Today the news is strikingly different. Minimally invasive laparoscopic surgical techniques have revolutionized surgical weight-loss procedures to the point where the majority of such operations can be performed in outpatient surgery facilities. Data from Western Bariatric Institute (*see Appendix A*), like that from many of the successful, high volume, high quality surgical centers, has shown a dramatic shift in recent years toward the outpatient arena. What was once a last-chance option in a (risky) operation is now an hour-long procedure that can change your life and have you home in time for dinner.

The term "laparoscopic" comes from the term *laparos*, meaning abdominal, and *oscopy* meaning using a camera to view what's inside the abdomen. Laparoscopic surgery is performed by inserting a long, thin camera (laparoscope) into the abdomen through tiny keyhole incisions so that complex surgical procedures can be performed without the traditional, larger, open incisions once required for weight-loss operations.

Types of Surgical Procedures

Among the top three surgical weight-loss procedures (in terms of popularity) are the LAGB, LRYGB and LSG.

LAGB (the LAP-BAND® Adjustable Banding System or the new REALIZE™ Band) allows a surgeon to place a flexible silicone band around the upper part of the stomach, effectively reducing the capacity of the stomach. The end result? The patient feels fuller faster, while eating less. A port under the skin allows the surgeon to inject or remove fluid from the band, making it tighter or looser.

LRYGB (laparoscopic Roux-en-Y gastric bypass) is a laparoscopic surgical technique that involves the creation of a small, 30-cc stomach pouch and a small outlet from the pouch directly into the small intestine, where nutrients are absorbed. With the majority of the stomach bypassed, and the pouch able to hold less volume than the stomach could, the person feels satisfied sooner and eats less.

LSG (laparoscopic sleeve gastrectomy) removes a large portion of the stomach. The remaining portion of stomach is formed into a long tube that is unable to enlarge or balloon up with food. The restriction reduces the amount a person can eat and causes satiety with less food. It can be performed as an outpatient procedure in centers that allow a 23-hour stay. LSG is a less complicated procedure than LRYGB and has fewer risks.

What is "Outpatient" Surgery?

Outpatient surgery usually means that the patient is expecting to come to the surgery center or hospital, undergo a surgical procedure, and return home the same day. In recent years, insurance plans and regulators have interpreted this to mean a release from the surgical facility within 24 hours.

As surgery has become less invasive, more procedures are being performed on an outpatient basis. In fact more operations of all kinds are performed on an outpatient basis than are performed on an inpatient basis (inpatient meaning there's a hospital stay involved).

With newer, less invasive surgical techniques and technology, even complex procedures such as orthopedic joint operations, spine procedures and even bariatric surgery can be performed with minimal stays.

For most surgeons and to most insurance plans, outpatient surgery means the patient undergoes surgery and returns home within 24 hours. In some cities and states, regulators have expanded the definition of "outpatient" to include certain facilities that allow patients to stay in the facility for up to 72 hours.

With the revolution of effective laparoscopic, minimally invasive weight-loss operations, LAGB and StomaphyX™ (a natural orifice procedure being developed to help people who have had previous weight-loss operations) procedures can usually be performed with a facility stay of a few hours. LSG may be performed with a 24 hour or shorter stay, and laparoscopic RYGB can be performed with a one- to two-night stay.

Such advances have been made across the fields of surgery (you're probably familiar with the term *arthroscopy,* which refers to operations performed on the joints using a camera inserted through small incisions). Such procedures traumatize the body less than open operations making it possible for patients to undergo even complex abdominal procedures with small incisions and minimal pain, discomfort and recovery time.

Another significant factor in the shift of bariatric surgery to outpatient facilities is the evolution toward perfection of two types of surgical weight-loss procedures. Laparoscopic improvements allow surgeons to perform both the laparoscopic Roux-en-Y gastric bypass (LRYGB, *see Chapter 2*) and the laparoscopic adjustable gastric band (LAGB, made popular by the LAP-BAND® from Allergan, Inc.; *see Chapter 2*). Both procedures can be performed by skilled laparoscopic surgeons in about an hour and in many cases require no hospital stay. A third procedure, known as the laparoscopic sleeve gastrectomy (LSG), is also emerging as an effective outpatient weight-loss procedure.

Generally, the LAGB procedure can be performed in 30 to 45 minutes with only 40 to 50 minutes of anesthesia time and a recovery time of only four to six hours in an outpatient surgery center. The laparoscopic RYGB usually requires an overnight stay as it is slightly more invasive, with more internal recovery time needed before patients are able to drink liquids (one of the indicators that a patient is ready to be discharged home). Also, there's a greater concern about complications with the laparoscopic Roux-en-Y procedure, which means surgeons prefer to have more patient observation time before discharge.

Twenty-five years ago most surgical procedures were performed in clinical hospital settings. Outpatient surgery centers began in the 1970s and proliferated in the 1980s, and today most U.S. operations are performed at outpatient surgery centers, with inpatient procedures actually on the decline. Outpatient procedures mean that the patient arrives, undergoes the operation and returns home on the same day or within 24 hours.

There are now 5,000 Medicare-certified outpatient surgery centers in the U.S., with more being built and coming online every month.

Outpatient surgery centers often have less red tape than full hospitals due to their specialization and expertise. They're also known for more flexibility with scheduling. Better still, outpatient surgery centers have superior safety records when compared to hospitals: an *Archives of Surgery* paper published in 2004 demonstrated the rate of serious complications and deaths following surgical procedures was significantly lower in outpatient surgical centers than in hospitals.[1] This is because the outpatient environment may have less serious hospital bacteria, because patients who can have procedures in outpatient settings have a lesser incidence of chronic illness, and because procedures performed in an outpatient setting are less invasive than those performed in a full hospital.

Outpatient surgery centers (also known as ASCs, ambulatory surgery centers) must comply with extensive inspections and certification programs in order to operate. Any outpatient surgery center serving Medicare beneficiaries must be certified by the United States Department of Health and Human Services in order to perform surgical procedures. This process involves compliance with an extensive set of standards and includes inspections and production of records and data. So, quality and safety are both factors that continue to drive the growth of outpatient centers. But most people would say the most important change leading to more outpatient weight-loss operations is simply that they work. Numerous long-term studies have shown the success of modern surgical weight-loss procedures in improving health, quality of life and longevity.[2-12]

If you're holding this book in your hands, chances are you or someone you love is or perhaps should be considering a surgical weight-loss procedure. It is my sincere hope that this book will help you understand the scope of outpatient surgical weight-loss procedures, their evolution and significant health benefits. An informed decision is always best.

Patient Story: David A.

Procedure: **LRYGB**
Weight lost: **205 pounds**

I chose weight-loss surgery for several reasons. I wanted to get my life healthy for my
loved ones, friends and especially myself.
The process prior to surgery wasn't bad.
There were some things I didn't want to do,
like blood work; I can't stand the sight of nee-
dles. But if you want something bad enough,
you'll do anything to get it! There were only
good things for the outcome. It's been a great
journey, and I wouldn't change anything! I just
wish I would have got my health back on track
a lot sooner in life!

The only concern I had prior to surgery was if
I was going to make it through the procedure.
I did, without any complications or problems,
thanks to my wonderful surgeon. Since surgery, I've had nothing but success. I've lost
about 75 percent of my excess body weight in
one year, and life's been great! I enjoy life and
look forward to each day. I'm very thankful
and grateful for this wonderful new tool and
my new life.

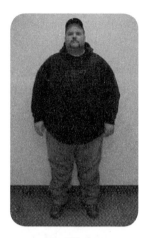

David before

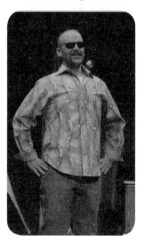

David after

Trends in Surgical Weight-Loss Procedures

The number of weight-loss surgeries performed in the United States is expected to be between 200,000 and nearly half a million by the year 2010.[13-16] I believe that is an underestimate, and some great technology and grim health statistics support my belief. The obesity epidemic in the U.S. is not letting up. Two-thirds of adult Americans are now considered overweight or obese; one-third of our children also fall into these categories.

We are living at a time when the solutions for serious weight loss are more effective than ever before and also markedly safer and less invasive. Many more people concerned with prevention of disease are considering minimally invasive weight-loss procedures before the onset of health problems that inevitably arise with weight gain.

The ravages of obesity are dramatic. Not only do overweight adults face shortened life spans but overweight children do as well. Excess weight carried over time causes dramatic increases in diabetes, high blood pressure, sleep disturbances, degenerative joint diseases, cancer, heart disease, asthma and a host of other complications.

Some people don't realize that the health problems that stem from the extra pounds occur with even modest weight gain. For

example, a study at Harvard shows being even moderately overweight increases the chance of developing type 2 diabetes (diabetes mellitus) sevenfold.[17] Age plays a role, as does genetic makeup,
in whether and when people develop problems such as high blood
pressure, asthma and diabetes. But even modest weight gain acts
as a powerfully detrimental force in bringing about unhealthy
conditions.

Simply stated, the number of Americans in need of serious and
effective weight-loss solutions easily exceeds 100 million people
annually.

Another reason I expect we're going to be seeing an increase in
weight-loss operations is the amount of information now getting
out to the public from reliable sources. Not only are you holding
in your hands a book on outpatient weight-loss surgery, but the
information is proliferating in other media as well.

With these highly effective and durable procedures now less
invasive and safer than ever before, a high percentage of patients
seeking weight-loss operations can undergo effective surgical weight loss with outpatient procedures.[18] And the advent of
even newer, even less invasive procedures is going to make getting healthy even more attractive. In 2008 the REALIZE™ Personal Banding Solution (similar to the LAP-BAND®) from Ethicon Endo-Surgery, Inc. (a division of Johnson & Johnson) was

marketed for the first time in the United States. The presence of two laparoscopic gastric band devices will catapult this type of procedure to new heights; I'm sure of it. And glad. For millions of people who have struggled with weight, these procedures will add years to their lives and remove years of suffering.

The effectiveness of modern bariatric procedures is extraordinary and results in stunning gains in life expectancy and health improvements. The procedures are swiftly moving from inpatient to outpatient settings, where patients experience less pain, more privacy and less time in hospital settings and recovery. I expect to see the frequency of outpatient surgical weight-loss procedures increase sharply as a trend in weight-loss surgery.

Our healthy future in this country depends on getting a grip on surging tides of obesity and weight gain. And until the complex root causes in our food supply, school policies and society are addressed, the need for effective weight-loss treatment will remain astronomical and continue to grow.

Weight-Loss Benefits

The first and most obvious benefit following surgical weight-loss procedures is, of course, weight loss. The change in appearance is often dramatic, and the health benefits are apparent almost at

once. Weight loss following modern minimally invasive outpatient bariatric surgical procedures is significant and long-lasting
in the vast majority of cases.

In order to take a look at modern bariatric surgery, I'd like to
examine the two most widely performed procedures: the laparoscopic adjustable gastric band (LAGB, such as the LAP-BAND®)
and the laparoscopic Roux-en-Y gastric bypass (LRYGB). Numerous long-term studies have identified the amount of weight lost
many years after LRYGB and LAGB.[5, 32] Most often, the weight
lost after the procedure is depicted as the percentage of excess
body weight lost.[19] What that means is if you weigh 200 pounds,
but your ideal body weight is 150 pounds, then your excess body
weight is 50 pounds. If you lost 40 pounds after the procedure,
then you would have lost 80 percent of excess body weight (40 is
80 percent of the 50 pounds you were over by).

Studies have shown that for the first two years post-surgery,
average weight loss from LRYGB is greater than weight loss from
LAGB. After the first two years, however, weight-loss outcomes
for both procedures are remarkably similar, according to several
studies. For example, a large Australian study examining the outcomes from both procedures found no significant difference in
long-term weight loss between the two procedures.[20]

Long-Term Results

In 2007 two articles appeared in the **New England Journal of Medicine** describing long-term follow-up studies after surgical weight-loss procedures.[5, 6] Both demonstrated dramatic positive results from operations, and both received a level of media coverage I hadn't seen in years. The front page of **The Wall Street Journal** described the studies and the findings, and many other national media outlets covered the news – surgical weight-loss procedures work: they reduce disease and health risks and increase longevity.

One of the studies **The Wall Street Journal** reported on, the Swedish Obese Subjects study, demonstrated a marked reduction in the 10-year mortality risk when an overweight patient undergoes a surgical weight-loss procedure. In the second study, overweight people in Utah were compared to patients who had undergone LRYGB procedures. The results confirmed again that surgical weight-loss procedures markedly improve long-term survival.[11]

Another study, this one published in 2005 by Maggard and colleagues, showed a consistently greater amount of weight loss observed for LRYGB when compared to LAGB at 12 months postoperative and then again at three years.[21] Both procedures result in profound, sustained, long-term weight loss and profound, well-documented physiological benefits and longevity (people who are healthier are simply apt to live longer).

It took a lot of doctors a lot of years to understand that being overweight or obese wasn't simply a matter of vanity or a cosmetic issue, but that being overweight was, in fact, unhealthy. The benefits of losing weight are almost instantaneous. Just as nearly every organ in the body is adversely affected by excessive weight, so is every organ system apt to benefit following weight loss – and all the more quickly following a surgical weight-loss procedure, when the weight is lost rapidly.

Many of the health complications caused by being overweight or obese can be markedly improved, or in some cases even resolved completely, by surgical weight-loss procedures. For younger people, who don't yet have elevated blood sugar or full diabetes or high blood pressure, weight-loss operations can prevent these dreaded health problems from ever beginning.

Following is a discussion of health conditions that can be prevented, significantly altered, improved or even cured following surgical weight-loss procedures. While all of these conditions can develop and exist independent of obesity, all of them can be caused by excessive weight, and all of them are exacerbated by excessive weight (and are therefore considered comorbid conditions). And in the vast majority of cases, these conditions can be improved or even resolved by weight loss. All of the following are dramatically improved by surgical weight-loss procedures:

Asthma and lung disease. Respiratory function, asthma and restrictive lung disease are improved by weight loss.[22]

Obstructive sleep apnea. Many studies have shown an alarming rise in the frequency and deadliness of sleep apnea in the U.S., primarily due to the obesity epidemic. Sleep apnea is a condition marked by snoring and periods when the person actually stops breathing because the soft tissues of the throat obstruct the passage of air. Virtually every study shows an early and profound reduction in sleep apnea in obese patients who undergo bariatric operations.[23-25] In a study in 2004, approximately 83 percent of patients with sleep apnea who underwent bariatric operations resolved the condition entirely without further need of external gear (such as a CPAP or nighttime supplemental oxygen).[25]

Hypertension and heart disease. Cardiac function and hypertension (high blood pressure) improve with weight loss. In one study, approximately 80 percent of patients involved found their high blood pressure either markedly improved or completely resolved after bariatric operations.[26]

Gastroesophageal reflux disease. Both LRYGB and the LAGB effectively separate the lower, acid-producing portion of the stomach from the esophagus so that the acid doesn't travel up into the esophagus and cause symptoms.[27]

Diabetes mellitus. Diabetes is currently at epidemic levels in the United States and other countries around the world. In the notably titled article, *Who Would Have Thought It? An Opera-*

tion is the Most Effective Treatment of Diabetes, Walter Poires followed 591 subjects who underwent LRYGB.[28] Of these, 94 had type 2 diabetes mellitus, and all but 11 saw their diabetes resolve completely post-operatively. Numerous other studies have documented the resolution of the condition following surgical weight-loss procedures.

Hepatic steatosis. This is a form of severe fatty deposits on the liver, a condition that leads to problems with liver function and the immune system. This leading cause of nonviral, non-alcohol-related cirrhosis improves markedly after surgical bariatric procedures.[29-31]

Polycystic Ovarian Syndrome (PCOS) and fertility. Obesity is a factor in infertility, as well as formation of ovarian cysts. Symptoms related to PCOS are improved in people who undergo bariatric operations.[32]

Other physical diseases and disorders. In addition, there exists a body of literature that links weight gain to:

» Degenerative joint disease;

» Pseudotumor Cerebri (a brain condition that causes severe headaches);

» Urinary incontinence; and

» **Venous stasis disease, a condition causing leg swelling and varicose veins.**

Depression and mental illness. A fascinating body of literature has emerged demonstrating that mental illness and obesity are, in fact, linked. A surprising amount of mental illness dissipates and resolves after a weight-loss surgical procedure, confirming that obesity and mental illness feed off each other.[33] This may be especially true of depression, the most common form of mental illness. Being depressed can lead to eating more and gaining weight, but it is also true that being severely overweight can lead to depression. So, once a person begins resolving the obesity, depression often lifts and self-esteem improves.

Quality of life. While difficult to measure in physiological terms, quality of life ranks among the most important measures of the success of any health intervention. If you're debating the value of surgical weight-loss procedures, ask yourself what you're missing in life. Is your weight stopping you from doing the things you want to do? Is fear of health complications due to weight causing you anxiety? And are complications from existing health issues taking away from your quality of life?

Numerous studies show the quality of life improves after a bariatric operation.[34, 35] But most people can figure this out for themselves. Experiencing reduction of pain in your joints and spine, watching diabetes melt away and having the doctor say this is the best shape you've been in for years all add up to a definite feeling of well-being.

Doctors tend to focus on cold numbers, such as mortality risk or odds ratios for experiencing a cardiac event. But for people who undergo weight-loss operations, what matters most may be the newfound ability to bend down and tie a shoe or pick up a child or run outside. It may be waking up in the morning without a feeling of dread or pain. For doctors in the field of bariatric surgery, it is probably the numerous and varied stories of improved quality of life that give us the energy and enthusiasm to keep trying to improve the care for our patients.

Survival. And the most important of all the health benefits of weight loss and surgical weight-loss procedures – life. Every study that has set out to measure the impact of bariatric procedures related to long-term survival has shown a striking advantage in favor of patients who undergo bariatric operations. Put as simply as possible: Seriously overweight people who undergo bariatric operations live longer, healthier lives.

Saving Lives

A large study of 6,000 morbidly obese patients in Canada by Christou et. al. compared those who underwent bariatric operations with those who did not.[36] After five years of study, those patients who underwent bariatric operations had an 89 percent reduction in mortality rates as compared with those who did not. In addition, patients who had bariatric operations had 50 percent fewer hospitalizations and significant reductions in cancer, cardiovascular, respiratory and infectious conditions. The same study did show, however, that surgical patients experienced higher rates of hospitalization for digestive or intestinal conditions.So, while the bariatric operations (primarily LRYGB in these patients) reduced the chances of heart attacks, pneumonia, cancer and death, the trade-off was an increase in one category of problems: those of the gastrointestinal tract. This doubtless stems from investigating potential problems with the gastric bypass or investigating symptoms such as vomiting that can arise from gastric bypass.

Are You a Candidate for Weight-Loss Surgery?

Surgical weight-loss procedures have come a long way in the last several decades. Not only have the procedures become much safer and much less invasive with the advent of laparoscopic surgery, but the surgical procedures themselves have come to be accepted in the medical field as having real health benefits rather than being viewed as simply cosmetic. The benefits to weight loss have been long-documented, and the benefits from weight-loss operations are now documented as well.

However, weight-loss operations are still surgical procedures, and not to be undertaken lightly. The risks of undergoing an operation must always be weighed against the benefits of that operation. That said, the health risks posed by being seriously overweight usually outweigh the inherent risks of modern surgical weight-loss procedures. But every case is different. The criteria used to select appropriate candidates for weight-loss operations were derived from a consensus conference statement put out by the National Institute of Health in 1991, and though a great deal has emerged and changed in the field since that time, little has changed for most centers with respect to their approach to choosing weight-loss operation candidates.

Since this book focuses on outpatient weight-loss surgery in particular, it doesn't cover the full range of topics covered in my upcoming comprehensive guide to surgical weight loss. However, let's touch briefly on what makes for a good candidate for surgical weight-loss procedures, then, more specifically, for outpatient weight-loss procedures.

	Height (ft)									
Weight (lbs)	4'9"	4'11"	5'1"	5'3"	5'5"	5'7"	5'9"	5'11"	6'1"	6'3"
154	33	31	29	27	26	24	23	22	20	19
165	36	33	31	29	28	26	24	23	22	21
176	38	36	33	31	29	28	26	25	23	22
187	40	38	35	33	31	29	28	26	25	24
198	43	40	37	35	33	31	29	28	26	25
209	45	42	40	37	35	33	31	29	28	26
220	48	44	42	39	37	35	33	31	29	28
231	50	47	44	41	39	36	34	32	31	29
243	52	49	46	43	40	38	36	34	32	30
254	55	51	48	45	42	40	38	35	34	32
265	57	53	50	47	44	42	39	37	35	33
276	59	56	52	49	46	43	41	39	37	35
287	62	58	54	51	48	45	42	40	38	36
298	64	60	56	53	50	47	44	42	39	37
309	67	62	58	55	51	48	46	43	41	39
320	69	64	60	57	53	50	47	45	42	40
331	71	67	62	59	55	52	49	46	44	42
342	74	69	65	61	57	54	51	48	45	43
353	76	71	67	63	59	55	52	49	47	44
364	78	73	69	64	61	57	54	51	48	46
375	81	76	71	66	62	59	56	52	50	47
386	83	78	73	68	64	61	57	54	51	48
397	86	80	75	70	66	62	59	56	53	50
408	88	82	77	72	68	64	60	57	54	51
419	90	84	79	74	70	66	62	59	56	53
430	93	87	81	76	72	67	64	60	57	54
441	95	89	85	78	73	69	65	62	58	55
452	98	91	85	80	75	71	67	63	60	57
463	100	93	87	82	77	73	69	65	61	58

Weight Category	*BMI*
Normal Weight	18.5 - 24.9
Overweight	25 - 29.9
Obesity	30 - 34.9
Severe Obesity	35 - 39.9
Morbid Obesity	≥40

Figure 1: *A* BMI *chart is a simplified way to determine your* BMI. *Simply find your height on the vertical chart, and then move horizontally until you find the column that expresses your weight.*

Ethicon Endo-Surgery, Inc., Allergan, Inc. and EndoGastric Solutions, Inc.

The criteria that determine candidates for weight-loss operations depend mainly on the calculation with which readers of this
book are probably most familiar: the Body Mass Index (BMI). BMI
is calculated from weight and height and is a reliable indicator of
body fat for most people.

For adults, BMI is calculated using the following formula:

weight (lb) / [height (in)]² x 703

» **Example: weight = 150 lbs, height = 5′5″ (65″)**

» **Calculation:** $[150 \div (65)^2] \times 703 = 24.96$ or:

» $150 \div (65 \times 65) \times 703 = 24.96$ or:

» $150 \div 4225 \times 703 = 24.96$

If you'd like to avoid doing the math yourself, online BMI calcu-
lators (such as mine at *www.SasseGuide.com*) perform the calculation for you. Or you may choose to use a BMI chart (*see Figure 1*).

While it wasn't intended to do so, the BMI has come to serve as
a guideline for physicians in determining if a patient is an appropriate candidate for a weight-loss operation. Generally if your BMI
is greater than 35 and you have health problems associated with
obesity (such as diabetes or high blood pressure), you are considered a candidate. Even in the absence of such comorbid conditions, if your BMI is greater than 40, you are a candidate. Increas-

ingly, experts believe people with BMIs greater than 30 are also candidates for the less-invasive weight-loss procedures that have emerged as outpatient surgery options described in this book. Studies show a real health benefit even in this mild to moderately obese group.[3]

Surgery Compared to Medical Weight Loss

In one study of the various weight-loss procedures available today, LAGB operations proved far more effective in treating obesity and the health conditions associated with it than multidisciplinary comprehensive medical weight-loss programs (medically supervised weight-loss programs, which included participation from physicians, physical trainers, nutritionists and other experts).[4] However, there is no official guideline or criteria for choosing a surgical weight-loss procedure. If you are considering a weight-loss operation, it will serve you to discuss your needs, wants and possible surgical outcomes with your physician and then make the choice that works for you.

Patient Criteria for Outpatient Surgery

Many outpatient centers have devised their own criteria to screen candidates for weight-loss operations, choosing only those in the low-risk categories, which is better for the centers and better for the patients. Choosing to perform procedures in only the low-risk categories is better for the centers because there are then fewer complications and hospital admissions over the course of the year. And since outpatient surgery centers have to report those statistics regularly, they want to show the best safety record possible. And of course the best safety record is exactly what patients want, too.

Following is the list we use at the Surgery Center of Reno. Our criteria have changed over time as we have performed thousands of weight-loss procedures. We have found that specific hard numbers (such as BMI) do not serve well as selection criteria, but rather each individual patient must be considered carefully and approved individually. Similar criteria are in use at other centers.

In order to undergo an outpatient weight-loss operation, a patient must have:

» **Approval for the outpatient procedure by the bariatric surgeon and anesthesiologist**

» **Approval by the outpatient center medical director (usually also an anesthesiologist)**

» **Approval by case conference committee if the BMI is more than 55**

» **No history of pulmonary hypertension**

» **An anesthesia risk factor classification of ASA III or less (the American Society of Anesthesiology classification system rates an individual's risk of surgical procedures from ASA I – lowest risk – to ASA V – highest risk)**

» **Sleep apnea well-controlled at home with the CPAP system or no sleep apnea present**

While there are no official criteria, rest assured that every surgeon, every surgical center and every insurance company has its
own interpretation of the data available on weight-loss surgery and
will apply its own criteria. For the most part, I have found that insurance companies typically require a BMI greater than 40, or a BMI
greater than 35 with comorbid conditions, whereas experienced
bariatric surgeons look at patients with a BMI of 30 and above as
candidates for weight-loss procedures, all the more so if comorbid
conditions are present. Which means there's a gray area between
what insurance companies see as warranting a life-changing operation and what physicians see as beneficial to a patient's health.

If you meet the surgeon's criteria or the surgery center's criteria
but not the criteria your insurance company considers valid, you
may want to consider paying out-of-pocket. This is a choice every
individual has to make for himself or herself, with the assistance
of a physician. (In *Chapter 4* we'll take a look at considerations for
those candidates for surgical weight-loss procedures who expect
to be paying out-of-pocket.)

Inpatient or Outpatient?

The decision to have an outpatient surgical weight-loss procedure
is a medical decision, ultimately best made by you and your physician together. Outpatient surgery centers follow different crite-

ria in determining which patients would benefit from outpatient procedures and which patients would be better served in-hospital. Outpatient surgery centers are usually not equipped to handle cases that require an inpatient hospital stay or cases that will involve actively managing complex medical problems.

So, if you have fairly severe medical problems like asthma or heart arrhythmias that require a lot of ongoing treatment and monitoring, and if your BMI is very high (say, greater than 55), and it makes it hard for you to breathe without supplemental oxygen, then you're probably looking at an inpatient hospital setting for your procedure. But it is best to discuss your individual case with your surgeon because sometimes even those conditions are handled effectively in the outpatient setting when the procedure is not very invasive.

Outpatient procedures are a better option for patients expected to undergo procedures with a minimum of complications and a very low chance of hospital admission. While I always hope there will be no complications at all, there is no way to reduce the risk to zero. I always prepare for the worst but plan for the best. Because patients undergoing outpatient weight-loss procedures stay, on average, only four to six hours in recovery in the center, they must be healthy enough to undergo the operation and anesthesia and still return home the same day.

If you have serious and active health considerations, especially those made worse by being severely overweight, then you are probably considered high risk for complications from anesthesia and a surgical procedure. The presence of severe sleep apnea, heart failure (or a related severe condition of the heart and lungs called pulmonary hypertension or *cor pulmonale*) and BMI greater than 55 have all been considered specific conditions that may preclude the outpatient setting. If this is the case, then for safety reasons your surgeon will likely recommend that the procedure be done at the hospital with at least an overnight stay.

Nonsurgical Weight-Loss Alternatives

Nonsurgical options in medical weight loss have evolved more gradually than the surgical options in the past two decades. Perhaps the biggest change has been in the attitude of physicians themselves, who have changed their perspective from that of weight loss being a vain, cosmetic goal that can be safely ignored in the majority of patients asking for medical assistance, to an understanding that weight loss for overweight or obese patients is crucial for improved health, easing of comorbid conditions and increased life spans.

Patient Story: Anita A.

Procedure: **LRYGB**
Weight lost: **205 pounds**

I didn't have any issues after surgery. In fact, I was very disciplined and committed to my exercise program and my new eating habits.

It was so rewarding to see the changes in my appearance and in my attitude. Each week I pushed myself to do something more challenging in my workout and try new things. I continued to write each day in my journal that I started.

I remember one day after working, driving by my work where there is a walking trail behind it, and it had a hill, and I remember saying to myself, "Wow, wouldn't it be cool to be able to one day climb up that and reach the top?" At that very moment, I made that a goal that within three months I would be climbing that hill, and I did! During this experience, I have discovered goals that I would set for myself and have achieved every one of them.

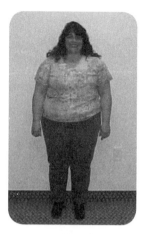

Anita before

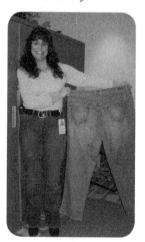

Anita after

Some of the nonsurgical options that have evolved since the 1980s include incremental improvements in techniques of behavior modification, physician-supervised medical weight-loss programs involving meal replacement bars and shakes, the use of improved and ever-safer prescription weight-loss medications and multidisciplinary weight-loss programs.

Medical (nonsurgical) weight-loss centers that can deliver multidisciplinary weight-loss programs – those programs that are physician-supervised and bring in other experts (from physical training coaches to life coaches to nutritionists) – have begun to emerge around the country, working with patients to develop state-of-the-art nonsurgical weight-loss techniques and treatment. I founded and serve as medical director of one of these nonsurgical centers, the International Metabolic Institute, or iMetabolic. iMetabolic centers, and other high-quality medically supervised weight-loss programs do achieve successes, but the successes often fall short of those achieved with surgical weight-loss procedures, especially in patients who are more severely overweight. Most studies examining medical (nonsurgical) treatment report that successful patients lose 5 to 10 percent of body weight when they adhere to medical weight-loss programs. Which is good, and even less invasive than the least invasive operation. And for many people with a BMI of 25 to 30, and some with a BMI of more than 30, it is exactly what they need to get healthy and lose weight.

For some people, medical weight-loss programs could be the answer they've been looking for to lose weight, keep it off and experience all the health benefits of doing so. But for many, these programs are only a step in the right direction and not the entire journey. Programs eventually must rely on patients being able to maintain self-control in a bewildering world of brightly lit advertisements for food in every newspaper and magazine, at every commercial break during television shows and in the popcorn-scented lobby of the local movie theater. Many of these programs utilize meal replacement shakes and prescription medicines, which are proven successful strategies in the short to mid term, but which may not be long-term solutions for weight loss for everyone.

Meal replacement bars and shakes work well for rapid weight-loss programs, especially those aimed at helping a patient lose weight before weight-loss surgery (*see Chapter 5 for further details*). But in a world of dizzying choices for meals virtually at our finger-tips, and in a person whose BMI has already climbed to more than 30, it's unlikely meal replacement bars or shakes are an option that will endure the test of time. More comprehensive medical weight-loss programs work to take that initial success and then build on it with behavior strategies and exercise to bring long-term success to those who are committed to change. This is exactly the strategy we have taken at iMetabolic, where the early successful weight loss of our induction programs using meal replacements are then sustained by long-term counseling, behavior change, coaching and support. Losing weight and keeping it off is not easy, though, and we employ a team of psychologists, in addition to life coaches, nutritionists, counselors, fitness trainers and physicians, to bring about the long-term change needed for sustained non-surgical weight loss. (Visit *www.iMetabolic.com* for more details on our commitment to medical weight loss.)

Unfortunately, few of the studies on nonsurgical medical weight-loss programs stretch beyond one year, at which point patients may well have started experiencing rebound weight gain. Surgical treatment studies normally report markedly greater weight loss and often follow patient progress for 10 or 15 years. Even with this discrepancy, studies that compare surgical and nonsurgical weight-loss treatment have shown that patients lose more weight and experience greater health benefits from surgical treatment.[37, 38]

Studies also show weight loss and improved health are more pronounced the heavier the individual was prior to beginning a program, an almost common-sense finding since the more over-weight a patient is the more likely the patient is to be suffering from comorbid conditions and the more weight the patient actually has to lose. And though heavier patients may show better numbers, the findings are well-documented beginning in patients with BMIs as low as 30.

Medically supervised weight-loss programs do not show the dramatic successes of weight-loss surgery, but those of us in the field are trying to improve those numbers as well. A medically supervised program can even be an excellent precursor to a surgical procedure. In fact, in our surgical weight-loss center, all patients lose weight first with medically-supervised programs for four to six weeks right before they undergo their operations. We have found that each patient loses weight, begins to learn better eating and exercise habits and becomes a better, safer surgical candidate with this approach.

Your choices are up to you, and only you can decide the best road for you. At the centers I lead, my staff and I work to provide the most comprehensive medical weight-loss programs in the world, with a dedicated team of physicians, psychologists, behavior experts, fitness coaches, nutrition experts and life and motivational coaches. For people committed to the long-term hard work involved, I think medically supervised weight loss is a great option, but it gets more difficult when the BMI has already risen to more than 30, and programs like ours at iMetabolic are tough to find in every city.

In the end, both nonsurgical and surgical programs play an important role helping overweight patients lose weight and improve their health.

» Calculate your BMI at *www.SasseGuide.com*

We know what we are,
but know not what we
may be.

– WILLIAM SHAKESPEARE

Food for Thought

» Weight-loss procedures have evolved since the early 1980s from full open operations to minimally invasive laparoscopic procedures that can often be performed at outpatient surgery centers.

» Because of the expertise and experience of surgeons and staff at outpatient surgical centers, weight-loss procedures have become increasingly safe over the last three decades.

» In 2007 approximately 200,000 weight-loss operations were performed in the U.S., the majority of which were LAGB or LRYGB procedures.

» Medical science now recognizes that the majority of weight-loss procedures are performed because of health risks or health problems rather than vanity.

» Medical conditions that can be dramatically improved or even totally reversed by weight-loss operations include asthma and lung disease, obstructive sleep apnea, hypertension and heart disease, gastroesophageal reflux disease, type 2 diabetes, hepatic steatosis, depression and mental illness, Polycystic Ovarian Syndrome and fertility problems.

» Seriously overweight people who undergo bariatric weight-loss operations live longer, healthier lives.

» If you are considering a weight-loss operation, you need to weigh the risks and benefits. Today's minimally invasive weight-loss operations are very safe, but there are always risks involved. The more you know, the better, so ask questions of your surgeon and his or her staff, and talk to anyone you know who has experienced the operation first hand or through the eyes of a loved one.

Change alone is eternal, perpetual, immortal.

– ARTHUR SCHOPENHAUER

2

Weighing Your Options

IN THE LAST three decades, increasing numbers of complex and invasive operations have moved from the confines of hospitals to the provenance of outpatient surgery settings – from orthopedics to spinal and neurosurgical procedures to gynecological, abdominal and general surgical procedures.

I've seen the changes myself, from both professional and personal points of view. During my training in the 1980s at the University of California, San Francisco, one of the premier university teaching facilities in the world, I witnessed and performed multiple gallbladder operations. At the time the new laparoscopic techniques with their small incisions were arriving on the scene. Patients underwent two- to three-hour surgical procedures, sometimes with two, three or even four surgeons, all of whom were just learning laparoscopic procedures. The hospital stay was two or three days long, taking the patient away from family and home, during which time a bewildering array of medical students and residents made rounds, poking, prodding and asking questions.

Patient Story: Teresa L.

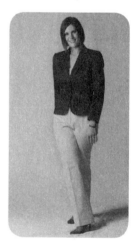

Procedure: **LRYGB**
Weight lost: **111 pounds**

I chose to have weight-loss surgery because I was unsuccessful with every conventional method tried. A friend and I actually went through the process together, which really helped.

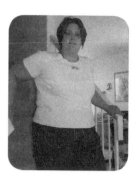

Teresa before

While learning about the surgery and going through the support sessions, you wonder if you are doing the right thing. You also try to figure out why you have to go to all the meetings and support groups. Let me tell you right now that it was worth it. You realize that there are others who used to be in the same place that you are in and that they went through this same process and look amazing now. It's hard to realize that you will look amazing one day but when you begin wearing sizes that have not been in your closet for over two decades, you realize that it can happen to you.

Teresa after

Fast forward to today, when gallbladder surgery is one of the most successful outpatient procedures in the field. Most of my patients scheduled for laparoscopic cholecystectomy (gall bladder removal) have the procedure at an outpatient surgery center. The surgery takes approximately 30 minutes to perform. Recovery time is two to three hours rather than two to three days, and patients return to their activities and active lives over the space of the next week, many returning to work during that timeframe, though possibly with some soreness and fatigue and some recovery work still left to do.

From a personal standpoint, when my own father had gallbladder attacks, he underwent a laparoscopic cholecystectomy on a Thursday, went home the same day and returned to work the following Monday, four days after surgery. This was unheard of when I was first learning about surgery.

Weight-loss surgery has changed just as dramatically as gallbladder surgery in the last 30 years. It is now possible to have life-changing surgery that can add years to your life and still return home on the same day.

Hospitals and outpatient surgery centers are only as safe as their employees and systems. This is good news when it comes to outpatient surgery centers where the volume of surgical procedures performed adds an edge of expertise. Working specifically in surgical procedures, these staff members are well-trained and experienced.[39]

But nothing is taken for granted. All outpatient surgery centers are required to have a plan in place for immediate transfer of any patient who develops complications. Many outpatient surgery centers are affiliated with large hospitals and medical centers and, in some cases, connected by underground tunnels, hallways or causeways. Transport, then, occurs instantly and seamlessly, so patients can enjoy the advantages of using an outpatient surgery center with the assurance of instant assistance from a full-service hospital if it becomes necessary.

The smaller size and sharper focus of outpatient surgery centers gives them added safety benefits as well. Outpatient surgery centers provide for less exposure to potential medical errors brought about by a large, overly-busy hospital bureaucracy and less exposure to the drug-resistant bacteria that populate hospitals throughout the United States.

So, knowing that outpatient surgical procedures are quite safe, the next question is:

Can You Really Have an Effective Weight-Loss Operation and be Home in Time for Tea?

Maybe not for tea, but almost undoubtedly in time for a protein-shake dinner. It's hard to imagine an operation as an outpatient procedure, something other than the week in a hospital with medical personnel overseeing and dictating your every move, but medical science has moved surgery to the point where more surgical procedures are performed in outpatient surgery centers than as inpatient procedures in hospitals.[40, 41]

It probably seems strange or incomprehensible, impossible, to believe that something as life-changing as surgical intervention for weight loss can take place in such a short time and still be effective. Part of this is the feeling that nothing can be attained in life without struggle – nothing comes easy.

An outpatient weight-loss operation is still an operation, an invasive procedure even if it is *minimally* invasive, with recovery time required, even if the recovery time is much shorter. There may even be the feeling that the weight didn't come on overnight, it came on over a long period of time, most likely over years or even decades – how can such a condition be reversed and changed in a single afternoon?

So, is it really possible to have a life-changing weight-loss procedure and be home the same day? Yes. Decades of research and technological advances have made such dreams reality.

	LRYGB	LAGB
No. of Patients	33	176
Female/Male	32/1	145/31
Mean Age	47 (±SD 8.9, range 29-69)	46 (±SD 10.9, range 21-69)
Mean Total O.R. Time (mins)	106 (±SD 27.4, range 45-167)	75 (±SD 36.3, range 55-179)

Figure 2: Features of same-day surgery/outpatient surgery of Western Bariatric Institute's patients at two outpatient surgery centers, from an initial study

In an early study of outpatient weight-loss surgery at Western Bariatric Institute, my colleagues and I reported on 194 patients who chose to undergo surgical weight-loss procedures at our outpatient surgery center. Approximately 90 percent of the patients who chose LAP-BAND® operations went home the same day, usually within four to six hours. One-hundred percent of the patients who had laparoscopic RYGB went home in less than 24 hours, after an overnight stay (*see Figure 2*).

Is a Surgical Outpatient Weight-Loss Procedure Right for You?

If you've struggled with weight gain for years, trying to keep it off or trying to lose it once it's found its way on, you know what a disheartening struggle weight-loss efforts can be. Maybe you've tried all the diets, bought into some fads and "medically proven" and celebrity-endorsed quick fixes. Maybe you've eaten only one food group or avoided another entirely, only to experience rebound weight gain.

And maybe you're tired of being tired, not having enough energy, feeling self-conscious about your weight or experiencing health problems because of it. If so, you are not alone, and you may be on the verge of finding answers to your problems. The answers aren't quick-fix solutions, nor do they involve effortless, instant weight loss. But the combination of modern, state-of-the-art out-patient weight-loss operations, combined with real commitment and quality medical advice is life-changing for most people. The solutions for serious weight loss and long-term health improvement are far more effective, and less invasive, than ever before.

A Word About Insurance and BMI

If your BMI is more than 30, you should be able to find a top-notch, highly qualified and skilled bariatric surgeon in the United States to take your case. A BMI of more than 30 means, in the eyes of many experts, you are an appropriate candidate, and the risks of surgery are less significant than the risks of not losing the weight. If your BMI calculates to 35 or more, you've got very good odds that standard commercial health insurance carriers will even cover the cost of the procedure. Of course, it's up to you, but in the event your health insurance carrier chooses not to cover the surgery, you may want to consider paying out-of-pocket. Take the time to fully understand all the potential costs involved, both short-term and long-term, as described in this book *(see Chapter 4 for a discussion of potential costs involved.)*

If you've been struggling with your weight, and you're tired of the constant fight and ready to move on to improved health and an improved life with a permanent, proactive solution, you may well be a candidate for a minimally to moderately invasive weight-loss operation. Modern outpatient weight-loss operations are not magical; they still require hard work to be successful. And like every procedure in medicine, there are risks and benefits to be weighed. But in most cases, with a minimum of risk, you can turn a losing uphill battle against weight gain into a battle you have proudly won.

Losing the weight and keeping it off is almost certainly the most important thing you can do for your health and longevity. Are you a candidate for outpatient weight-loss surgery?

Laparoscopic Adjustable Gastric Band (LAGB) Procedure

The laparoscopic adjustable gastric band (LAGB, using the LAP-BAND® or REALIZE™ Band) procedure is by far the most common and popular outpatient weight-loss procedure, worldwide, available today. The idea behind LAGB is almost as simple as tightening your belt, only in this instance the belt is internal. During the LAGB procedure a soft silicon polymer band is placed around the upper stomach and positioned so that a medical professional can adjust and tighten the band periodically as weight loss occurs (*see Figures 3 and 4*).

The technical result is that after the procedure a person with an adjustable gastric band experiences a state of satiety, feeling full through mechanisms that may be hormonal, stimulated by body tissues, or mechanical and psychological.[7] The procedure may trigger weight loss in patients in several different ways: by changing the body's hormones, by direct pressure on the stomach, which signals the brain to eat less, as well as other nerve-assisted mechanisms.

LAGB also has that belt-tightening effect: it produces weight loss through a restrictive mechanism, by making the stomach smaller and unable to hold as much in one sitting, and thereby limits the size of meals and amount of calories that can be consumed. As weight loss occurs, physicians can tighten the gastric band through an injection of saline through a small port inserted beneath the skin during

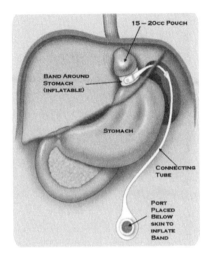

Figure 3: Laparoscopic adjustable gastric band. The procedure consists of two parts: first inserting the band around the upper stomach and, second, placing an access port under the skin of the abdominal wall.

the LAGB procedure. The saline makes the band thicker and therefore tighter, which allows patients to continue achieving satiety and weight loss over time.

The LAGB has significant advantages that have made it the procedure of choice in Australia and many countries in Europe. It has taken longer to catch on in the United States because it took longer to go through the FDA approval process. However, while the FDA was doing its job, surgeons in the U.S. continued to do theirs, changing and improving upon other surgical weight-loss techniques, most notably the LRYGB procedure.

Hormones and Hunger

Hormones are chemicals secreted by the tissues of the body's organs that travel through the bloodstream to exert an effect on another part of the body. For example, adrenaline is a hormone produced by the adrenal glands in response to fear or excitement. Adrenaline travels through the bloodstream causing the heart to beat faster and the blood pressure to rise. Adrenaline even causes our irises to open wider and let in more light to the eyes, to help us flee or fight. We are just beginning to understand the hormones produced by the stomach and other digestive organs, and how these hormones affect our sense of hunger and satiety. We think that after LAGB surgery, changes in these hormones may occur, so that the signals traveling to the brain cause a reduction in the level of hunger we experience. Some of the important hormones involved in hunger are ghrelin, insulin and leptin, but many more are waiting to be discovered and named.

The body communicates from organ to organ using nerves and with hormones that travel through the bloodstream. A complex web of such nerves exists between the brain and the digestive organs of the body. It is believed that some of these nerves carry signals that tell our brains we are full when our stomachs are distended, a phenomenon called "proprioception." Placing the band on the stomach, or performing other weight-loss operations, may induce just this type of signaling that reduces hunger and contributes to the overall, long-term weight loss.

LAGB is a minimally invasive procedure because no gut tissues or organs are removed, stapled or redirected. It is commonly performed as an outpatient procedure, with the patient returning home the same day as surgery.

LAGB procedures are also reversible, an attractive feature when we consider the pace of change in a field that has seen numerous revolutions toward less invasive and more successful interventions.

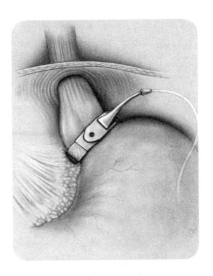

Mortality risks for LAGB have generally ranged from 0 to 0.1 percent, lower than that of LRYGB, though experienced centers such as where I work report LRYGB mortality rates of 0.1 to 0.2 percent.[42-45]

Figure 4: Laparoscopic adjustable gastric band. Close-up illustration of the gastric band placed around the upper part of the stomach. The band adjusts or tightens when the cuff is inflated with saline solutions, administered through the access port (not depicted).

As you can see from the following figure, more and more Americans are undergoing weight-loss surgery each year. In 2007, more than 200,000 Americans underwent weight-loss operations, nearly all of them LAP-BAND® or gastric bypass procedures. (*For a discussion on which laparoscopic band might work for you, see Appendix D.*)

Laparoscopic Roux-en-Y Gastric Bypass (LRYGB) Procedure

Laparoscopic Roux-en-Y gastric bypass (LRYGB) is a more complicated procedure than LAGB. It involves creation of a small, 30-cc, stomach pouch, and an outlet from the pouch directly into the upper intestine, where nutrients are absorbed (*see Figures 5 and 6*). By doing this, the majority of the stomach is bypassed, and the pouch, which has less volume than the stomach did, fills more quickly and makes the patient feel full and eat less.

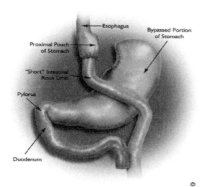

Figure 5: Laparoscopic Roux-en-Y gastric bypass. The small stomach pouch is created and separated from the rest of the stomach. Then the portion of the small intestine called the Roux limb is brought up and connected to the stomach pouch.

Gastric bypass also intentionally reduces the absorption of some nutrients into the bloodstream. This is because the enzymes that allow our bodies to break down and digest nutrients come from the stomach and the pancreas. After bypass, these enzymes travel downstream and don't come into contact with the food eaten until later in the digestive process. Usually the surgeon creates a length of intestine of around 100 cm, although sometimes we create longer segments for more severely obese patients.

This first part of the intestine is not absorbing nutrients as it would normally because there are no digestive stomach and pancreatic enzymes present over the length of the first 100 cm. After that distance of intestinal length, the enzymes join the digesting food, and normal absorption of nutrients begins in the remaining length of the intestine.

Researchers believe one reason LRYGB works for so many people is that the restrictive nature of the pouch limits the amount of food that can be eaten – there simply isn't room in the stomach any longer to allow the person to overeat. The same kinds of hormonal, psychological and nerve-mediated weight-loss signals may be at work as we described for LAGB. In addition, malabsorption causes fewer of the calories eaten to actually be absorbed into the bloodstream and into the body to be burned or stored as fat.

Many patients who undergo LRYGB experience a phenomenon known as "dumping syndrome," which is about as unpleasant as it sounds. Dumping syndrome results in unpleasant flushing, cardiac palpitations and nausea when the patient eats foods rich in carbohydrates (such as desserts). While these side effects are unpleasant and can continue to be present as late as 10 years after the operation, they also work as negative reinforcement, a kind of a behavioral conditioning technique that backs up medical advice to avoid carbohydrates after undergoing the LRYGB procedure. On the plus side, many studies have shown long-term sustained weight loss from 49 to 95 percent of excess preoperative body weight.[36]

A variation on the LRYGB procedure allows for a longer bypass to be created with a 150-cm or 200-cm Roux limb (the part of the intestine brought up and connected to the stomach pouch), which may increase weight loss in patients with higher than average BMI. The greater weight-loss results from even more calories passing through the intestine without being absorbed into the bloodstream.

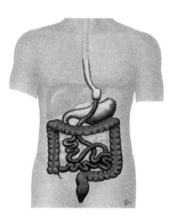

Figure 6: Image of the completed laparoscopic Roux-en-Y gastric bypass procedure. This illustration depicts the entire abdominal and intestinal anatomy after completion of the procedure.

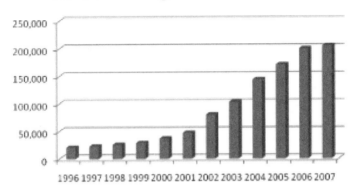

Figure 7: Bariatric surgery in the U.S. The numbers along the side represent annual procedures; the numbers along the bottom represent the year.

LRYGB is not a new procedure. It's been with us for decades. The name comes from a French surgeon named Roux and the "Y" configuration that results when the intestine is brought up to connect to the stomach pouch.[47] While it's not the newest procedure in our arsenal of weight-loss solutions, the procedure has come a long way since the 1960s and 70s and even since the 1980s and 90s when the operation was still usually performed with an open technique. Some modifications have taken place, such as improved knowledge of the ideal stomach pouch size, ideal length of the Roux limb and better stapling techniques. Now, with the minimally invasive, or laparoscopic, technique, many surgeons favor it as the state-of-the-art weight-loss operation with the best long-term results, especially for more seriously overweight patients.

In my outpatient surgery practice, I tend to keep patients overnight if they opt for the LRYGB. However, LRYGB can be performed as outpatient weight-loss surgery under special circumstances – if the patient is a safe candidate, without serious heart or lung problems, and motivated to walk, move and recover quickly.

Laparoscopic Sleeve Gastrectomy Procedure

A third procedure emerging on the minimally invasive weight-loss surgery scene is called the laparoscopic sleeve gastrectomy (LSG). The procedure can be performed as outpatient surgery and involves removing a large portion of the stomach. The remaining portion of the stomach is formed into a long tube that is unable to enlarge or balloon up with food. There's not much long-term data on this procedure yet, but so far it appears effective in producing weight loss by restricting the amount a person can eat and creating a sense of fullness. It can be performed as an outpatient procedure in selected cases in centers that allow a 23-hour stay. Sleeve gastrectomy has the advantage of being a less complicated or difficult procedure than the LRYGB, with fewer risks.

LSG is becoming recognized as another good outpatient weight-loss surgical procedure for several reasons. First, it can be performed safely in about an hour with a laparoscopic approach, like the other procedures. Since it does not involve an intestinal connection, there's no problem of impaired absorption of vitamins and minerals, or any of the risks caused by the intricate work required in the LRYGB. As a straightforward removal of a portion of the stomach, the LSG offers a simplicity that makes it work well in the outpatient setting. Although concerns persist that patients will stretch out the stomach over time, many in this field believe LSG will play a role for years to come.

Emerging Technologies

We've already examined two common weight-loss surgical procedures, the LAGB and the LRYGB, and a less common one, the LSG. LAGB is routinely performed in outpatient procedures, while LRYGB and, increasingly, LSG, can be outpatient procedures under special circumstances.

New technologies are evolving to meet the needs of society's ongoing search for improved health. Surgeons and surgical technology companies have continued to make advances in surgical instrumentation and techniques, making more procedures available, decreasing the invasiveness of procedures and increasing safety. Laparoscopic techniques moved surgical science light years ahead in increasing safety over the old, open-surgery techniques. Now some researchers believe even the minimally invasive laparoscopic procedures will give way to procedures that require no incisions whatsoever.

The Intragastric Balloon. Is that still surgery, you ask? Surgery without incisions sounds like magic. Not quite. But it is a more natural approach to surgical technique, utilizing the body's existing orifices. The procedure involves passing an endoscope down the mouth and esophagus, into the stomach to plant a large balloon there (*see Figure 8*). The balloon occupies space in the stomach, simulating a feeling of fullness and decreasing hunger. So far,

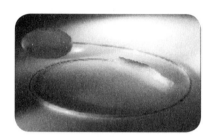

Figure 8: Intragastric Balloon. The balloon is placed inside the stomach and released to stay there, producing a sense of fullness or satiety.

results are mixed on this surgical procedure – patient weight-loss and satisfaction track records aren't as strong as they could be.[48-50] It remains to be seen whether or not the intragastric balloon will come into greater use in the future.

StomaphyX.™ Another natural orifice procedure being developed involves passing an endoscope and then using some novel technology to suture or plicate the stomach and create small pouches or valves. Currently, it is only useful for people who have already had a previous weight-loss stomach operation, such as LRYGB or LSG, but failed to lose adequate amounts of weight or who are regaining weight. The nifty thing about StomaphyX™ is that it is a way of performing stomach surgery without an incision; all the work is done via a tube passed down the mouth and into the stomach.

This procedure actually involves redesigning the stomach into a better functioning organ. A stretched stomach pouch can be re-tightened with this technique, and the sense of restriction once again restored. Changing the stomach's outflow design means patients once again experience stomach restriction, feel more satisfaction and less hunger, which should result in eating less and continued weight loss (*Figure 9*). Approved by the FDA in 2007, this device is gaining popularity among sophisticated bariatric surgeons who view it as an alternative to a more complex or invasive revision procedure.

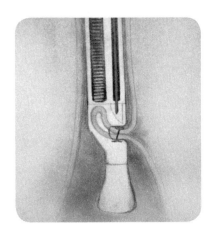

Figure 9: StomaphyX.™ In this procedure a soft tube, a type of sophisticated lighted endoscope, is passed down the mouth and esophagus into the stomach. No incisions are made. The stomach pouch can be tightened by placing internal fasteners in the stomach tissue.

People who experience severe reflux or heartburn may benefit from the StomaphyX™ procedure (and the related device called EsophyX™)[51] because the tissues of the stomach can be tightened, thus restoring a natural valve that blocks stomach contents from refluxing up into the esophagus. The procedure may also help with people who experience severe dumping syndrome related to rapid passage of food from the stomach pouch directly out into the intestine after gastric bypass. By re-tightening and shrinking the stomach pouch and the outflow area, the dumping may slow down.

Other companies are working on similar technology. Ethicon and other companies are developing products that involve placing internal stomach sutures.

Beyond the use of natural orifice surgery in weight-loss procedures, the techniques are being used for other surgical procedures that currently employ laparoscopic techniques. For example, pioneering surgeons in this field can remove a gallbladder or appendix without external incisions other than one to place a camera. Other incisions are made to maneuver the camera through internal organs. This kind of surgery is called NOTES (Natural Orifice Transluminal Endoscopic Surgery).[52]

One last technologically advanced type of weight-loss surgery has been in use for several years now – gastric pacemaking. This procedure involves placing electrodes on the stomach wall, modifying the electrical signaling in the stomach to create a sense of fullness or satiety. Modest success has been achieved, but the idea hasn't really caught on with either surgeons or patients.[53-55]

Change does not necessarily assure progress, but progress implacably requires change. Education is essential to change, for education creates both new wants and the ability to satisfy them.

– HENRY STEELE COMMAGER

Food for Thought

» In the last 30 years, increasing numbers of complex and invasive surgical procedures have changed from open procedures requiring in-hospital stays to minimally invasive laparoscopic procedures performed in outpatient surgery centers, with patients able to return home the same day.

» The volume of surgical procedures performed at outpatient surgery centers gives staff there an edge from expertise. Procedures are usually safer, but always do your homework and investigate everything when contemplating undergoing surgery.

» While most patients undergoing surgical procedures in an outpatient center are healthier than patients who need to be in-hospital, still all outpatient centers have a contingency plan for moving patients to a hospital within minutes if complications occur.

» It is now possible to have a life-changing weight-loss surgical procedure and be home in time for dinner.

» The laparoscopic adjustable gastric band (LAGB, using the LAP-BAND® or REALIZE™ band) procedure is by far the most common and popular outpatient weight-loss procedure, worldwide, available today.

» The LAGB works essentially like tightening your belt: The soft, flexible silicon band placed around the upper stomach creates a feeling of being full after eating less, encouraging weight loss and preventing overeating.

» The laparoscopic Roux-en-Y gastric bypass (LRYGB) involves creation of a small stomach pouch that allows nutrients to bypass the majority of the stomach. The pouch, being smaller than the stomach, creates a feeling of fullness sooner and with less food consumed, and also reduces some of the absorption of nutrients.

» The third minimally invasive weight-loss procedure is the laparoscopic sleeve gastrectomy (LSG), which involves removing a portion of the stomach and leaving a long tube that is unable to fill up with large amounts of food.

» Other new, less commonly used weight-loss techniques include the intragastric balloon, StomaphyX™, Ethicon's cinch device (which involves internal stomach sutures) and gastric pacemaking, which involves placing electrodes on the stomach wall and modifying the electrical signaling in the stomach to create a sense of fullness or satiety.

It is not the strongest of the species that survives, nor the most intelligent,

but the one most responsive to change.

– Charles Darwin

3

Risk and Reward

SURGICAL WEIGHT-LOSS PROCEDURES are safer today than they ever have been before. But I cannot emphasize enough how important it is to understand the very real risks of undergoing a surgical procedure and the need to compare those to the tremendous benefits and improvements to health and to quality of life that may come from substantial long-term weight loss. Any significant life-changing decision should include an understanding of both the positives and negatives, both the upsides and the downsides, both risks and benefits. There is no such thing as too much information when it comes to deciding on whether or not to have a surgical procedure, take a prescription medicine or pursue a health treatment strategy. Read everything you can get your hands on. Talk to everyone you know who may have undergone the same operation or had a friend or loved one who did. Get second opinions.

Keep in mind there is a body of data showing that, for those patients with significant health risks and a BMI of more than 35, *not* undergoing a surgical weight-loss procedure is more dangerous than doing so, even with the attendant risks.

The Evolution of Gastric Banding

Open vertical banded gastroplasty gained popularity in the 1970s as an open abdominal procedure involving placement of a nonadjustable, firm silicon band around the upper stomach **(see Figure 10)**. It was successful in producing weight loss, and was still being recommended at the time of the NIH Consensus Conference in 1991. However, some problems arose with band erosion into the stomach tissues, and the long-term weight-loss results were disappointing.[56, 57]

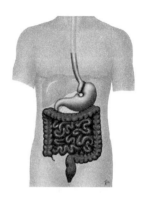

Figure 10: Vertical banded gastroplasty was popular in the 1970s and 80s.

Beginning with the Swedish band (now being released in the U.S. as the REALIZE™ Band), and continuing to the LAP-BAND®, surgeons and engineers created a softer, adjustable band that had fewer problems and could be placed laparoscopically **(see Figure 11)**. The new generation of bands can be adjusted over time, and the long-term weight loss, as a result, is markedly better.

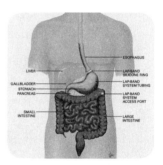

Figure 11: Placement of the LAP-BAND® during the LAGB surgical procedure.

The 1991 NIH Consensus Conference statement on obesity concluded the question came down to risk vs. benefit: Was it riskier in the long term for a person to remain seriously overweight, even morbidly obese, and not undergo a surgical weight-loss procedure, or was it better in the long run and less risky overall to undergo a major open operation? The conclusion at the time took into account data that focused on open operations with all their risks, rather than today's much safer, minimally invasive procedures. At the time the consensus was drafted, the mortality rate as evidenced by major studies from the 1980s exceeded 5 percent for the open procedures. *Still, in light of those facts, the consensus was that despite the risks of the weight-loss operations available at that time, the risks of remaining seriously overweight, in fact, exceeded the risks of going through the operation.*

It says a lot about the high risks of being seriously overweight that such a conclusion could be reached in an era when the operations being offered were so much less safe and so much more invasive than the procedures available today.

The innovations and technology that have marked the revolution in weight-loss surgery have not changed a simple idea. What has changed is the level of safety. Many of the weight-loss operations performed today are the same in theory as they were in the 1980s and 90s but with modifications that have enhanced effectiveness while reducing risks. For example, the open Roux-en-Y gastric bypass has undergone several minor modifications (changes in stomach pouch size, use of newer staplers, adjustments of the length of the intestine bypassed), and one revolutionary change (the switch to laparoscopic, minimally invasive technique). The long-term weight-loss results are the same or better in magnitude than they were 30 years ago, but the safety record is astronomically improved.

Today, in the hands of a skilled surgeon at a nationally recognized Center of Excellence, or at one of many other high-quality, high-volume centers, the mortality risk for undergoing a minimally invasive bariatric operation ought to be less than one in 1,000. Think of it: Only 20 years ago that same operation carried a mortality risk perhaps as great as one in 20 and now the risk is less than one in 1,000, and, in some cases, published risks from high volume centers such as where I work are below even that.[58-60]

Experience Matters

Before we go into detail about the types of risks associated with each type of weight-loss surgical procedure, I want to emphasize that these risk percentages apply only to people undergoing procedures performed by experienced, well-trained bariatric surgeons. I can't emphasize enough how important it is to seek out an experienced, well-trained surgeon with a proven track record before undergoing such an important step.

Data on many types of complex surgical procedures, such as cardiac bypass and pancreatic resections, shows that complication and mortality risks are far lower and results far better in the hands of well-trained, experienced surgeons. Just as an outpatient surgery center will often have a better track record for safety due to its focus on one thing – surgery – than a general hospital tasked with caring for any and every contingency, so a surgeon who focuses on specific operations and has trained for and performed many of the same operations will have a better safety and results record (results are measured by the lack of complications from procedures performed and success of weight loss following the procedure).

Risks of Outpatient Surgical Weight-Loss Procedures

The increase in the number of bariatric surgical procedures performed in the United States has risen at the same time obesity rates have risen among the population.

During the same period of time the related risks of outpatient weight-loss operations have fallen in proportion to the numbers of procedures performed. The more experienced surgeons become and the more weight-loss operations are performed, the safer the procedures become.

Centers of Excellence

The American Society of Metabolic and Bariatric Surgery acknowledges Centers of Excellence in bariatric surgery through the arm of the organization known as Surgical Review Corporation, or SRC. The SRC has undertaken the noble process of certifying programs throughout the country by meticulously reviewing data submitted by the programs and the hospitals or surgery centers and then by performing site visits and inspections. The effort is meant to provide standards of reporting and standards of quality that anyone can rely upon when selecting a bariatric surgeon.

Confusingly, another surgical organization, the American College of Surgeons, also started a certification process for bariatric Centers of Excellence, with much the same objectives. For political reasons, the two organizations were unable to work together to maintain only one certifying body.

Even more confusing and, from some points of view, bizarre, some insurance plans, such as Blue Cross of California, have undertaken their own effort to certify programs, called Centers of Expertise, which of course do not recognize the Centers of Excellence identified by the above two surgical organizations.

Are the COEs really **excellent** or **expert**? Probably. Are there excellent bariatric surgeons who are not members of COEs? Undoubtedly.

For the surgeon and the surgeon's practice, COE designation proves expensive, time-consuming and cumbersome to apply for from even one of these entities, let alone three or more. The process systematically favors larger institutional programs that are usually university-based because of the unusually large investment of time and resources to comply with the application process and the data-reporting requirements. These do not necessarily guarantee the best surgeons or the best programs; these entities may simply have the staff and budget to undertake the bureaucratic effort. Which means that checking the Centers of Excellence Web site (http://www.surgicalreview.org) is a good first step when searching for a surgeon, but it's not the only step. The site can't tell you if a surgeon is careful or that all the results of the practice have been excellent. It can tell you if a surgeon and a practice have worked hard to complete an extensive application process, made sure all the equipment is state-of-the-art and have established a good process for following and reporting surgical outcomes.

For my part, I didn't mind. I didn't mind taking the time and energy to complete the COE application because Western Bariatric Institute's practice had already put in place nearly all of the required elements, and I felt it would help potential patients recognize that we were committed to our patients' success.

In the future, COEs may be the only centers that insurers will reimburse. On the other hand, surgical practices that find the process expensive and cumbersome may opt out and appeal directly to consumers based on their local excellent track records. Hopefully, the COE process will serve patients well by raising the standards of the field and insisting on certain minimums of experience and proper equipment and outcomes so that safety and weight-loss success will be maximized.

Mortality risk for bariatric surgical procedures has declined sharply since the 1970s and 80s. If you're remembering all the risks related to weight-loss operations, likely you're remembering the early days of the procedures, when mortality rates of 10 percent were not uncommon. Bariatric operations are much less dangerous now. Studies have appeared over the last two decades that chronicle the falling risk and mortality rates. A study covering the years 1987 to 2001 and including more than 3,300 bariatric procedures in Washington State showed an overall 30-day mortality rate of 1.9 percent.[61] A separate study of more than 16,000 LRYGB procedures in California showed a mortality rate of 0.3 percent.[62] As the years have passed, the reported mortality rates have continued to drop.

For LAGB procedures, the risk of death varies from 0 to 0.3 percent depending on the study, though most large studies report rates well below 0.1 percent. A systematic review in Australia found LAGB approximately tenfold safer than gastric bypass in terms of the 30-day mortality risk.[63, 64]

Other studies have contradicted this wide disparity in safety between the two procedures. For while both procedures have become very safe and effective with experienced surgeons, there exists a certain low level of baseline risk that stems from a seriously overweight patient undergoing an operation of any kind.

What this means in human terms, rather than in stark numbers of mortality, is this: For every 1,000 patients who undergo LAGB surgical procedures, one may face complications that result in death.

Consider this fact for the sake of comparison: In any given year, a person with a BMI of more than 40 faces a substantially higher risk of death, around a 1 to 2 percent chance, just from the strain on the heart and lungs and the complications of diabetes, blood clots and other conditions created or exacerbated by the extra pounds.[65, 66]

The American meta-analysis (a study that combines and analyzes results from many studies, performed to reach broader conclusions than individual studies alone) found no significant difference in mortality between the gastric bypass and the LAGB procedures.[21] What studies did show was that the more experienced the surgeon, the lower the risk of mortality and serious complications.[61]

Another study also noted that the percentage of risk drops with the experience of the surgeon: Surgeons who have performed 20 procedures operate with a 6 percent mortality risk; surgeons who have performed more than 250 procedures have a risk of virtually zero percent.[27]

At Western Bariatric Institute, we've seen our own data confirm these findings. Among our more than 3,000 cases, the overall 30-day mortality risk since the practice was started is less than 0.2 percent. In our practice we perform primarily LRYGB procedures and a lesser number of LAGB procedures. The statistics at our center corroborate what is reported in the literature. The drop in mortality rates is occurring for many reasons: better systems in place to prevent errors, better patient selection and evaluation prior to surgery, preoperative weight loss and risk reduction, improved experience of the nursing, anesthesia and surgical staff, and better patient education.

Postoperative Nausea and Vomiting

Probably the most frequent adverse event reported by patients undergoing any kind of operation, including bariatric procedure, is postoperative nausea and vomiting. Whether it is caused by the combination of the anesthetic drugs used during operations or the laparoscopy or the manipulation of the stomach itself, the result is a significant number of people with some postoperative nausea.

For many people, this is fairly mild and goes away within a few hours to a day. In other people it is not present at all. In very rare cases there may be some more serious cause for postoperative nausea and vomiting, such as a blockage of the intestine. Generally if the symptoms persist more than a few days the surgeon will begin looking for other potential causes with X-ray studies, but generally speaking, surgeons look first at the narcotic pain medications, anesthetics and other drugs, including antibiotics, which can cause nausea for some people.

Vomiting is not usually dangerous and will almost never harm the incisions of a laparoscopic procedure. But it is unpleasant, even painful, and therefore my staff and I work to avoid it in all our patients.

Sometimes when the gastric pouch is fairly small and the anastomosis (where the stomach is connected to the intestine) is fairly snug, people experience some nausea and regurgitation or vomiting early in the first few days or weeks after the procedure as they begin eating and drinking again. This is reasonably common and is nothing to be alarmed about as long as the patient is able to continue drinking and stay hydrated. The condition, in general, should improve over time. If symptoms appear to be worsening instead of improving over the course of two or three days, or if other, more serious, symptoms (such as high fevers and shaking or chills) and serious pain occur, a call to the surgeon and a trip to the physician's office or hospital will be required.

Heart, Lung, Kidney and Other Organ Dysfunction and Complications

Complications that arise with the major organs either during or after operations are generally due to underlying conditions, sometimes undiagnosed, from which seriously overweight people may suffer. And while it may seem as if a health condition important enough to cause serious complications with organs during or after weight-loss procedures should have been easily diagnosed before surgery, that isn't always the case.

For example, a high percentage of people who are seriously overweight have undiagnosed hypertension and hypertensive heart disease. Many people have not had their blood pressure checked or had a physical exam or had blood tests of the kidney function even taken, for years. In addition, blood pressure readings can vary for a number of reasons – people may be nervous in a medical setting so the readings go up and aren't accounted for because of the setting in which the reading was attained. People can be diagnosed with hypertension just because they are always nervous when they're in a doctor's office and, as a result, "hypertensive," when really throughout the day, when they're not around anyone from the medical community, their blood pressure is in the normal range. Blood pressure readings also vary from day to day, week to week, before and after meals and depending on the level of hydration in the body.

Because of the variations between readings, people can go for years without knowing they've got high blood pressure, and all the while the condition worsens simply because readings were taken at times when blood pressure was lower than average.

Nonetheless, it is quite common for a person to have suffered the effects of hypertension with slow but steady damage to the heart, arteries and blood vessels, and brain for years prior to coming in for a weight-loss procedure. The same can be said for damage to the kidneys and damage to the lungs. Just as a long-term smoker can often have undiagnosed or unrecognized emphysema, a person with long-term obesity can have unrecognized damage or dysfunction of the lungs, kidneys and other organs simply as a result of the years of extra weight.

Previously undetected damage to the organs can become a problem postoperatively when a patient is apt to be in a weakened condition and more vulnerable to illness, infection and organ dysfunction as a result of an operation and having been under anesthesia. Experienced bariatric staff are aware of these potential issues and are always on the lookout for some kind of organ dysfunction during the postoperative period. Normally, my staff and I test for these types of events with laboratory tests before and after weight-loss surgery.

Cardiac arrhythmias (irregular heartbeat) and postoperative hypoxia (low levels of oxygen in the blood) are two of the most common postoperative problems.

Usually, my staff and I are able to anticipate undiagnosed serious heart disease, and we test for this in the preoperative stage, so we don't often get many surprises of serious postoperative heart problems. However, even a person who has passed a preoperative stress test with flying colors can, on rare occasion, experience a serious postoperative heart attack. Likewise, a person who generally doesn't have exceptional shortness of breath during everyday life may experience serious shortness of breath or even develop postoperative pneumonia or hypoxia after undergoing an operation.

These complications are more common after open procedures than they are following laparoscopic procedures. In particular, pulmonary (lung) complications are much less apt to occur after a laparoscopic procedure than an open procedure because the pain and the cutting of the abdominal wall in open procedures is so much less invasive in the laparoscopy procedures.[67-69]

Blood Clots

Blood clots remain an important potential complication after any type of surgical procedure, including those used for weight loss. People who are seriously overweight are – you guessed it – at an increased risk of developing blood clots over and above that of the standard normal-weight patient.

Blood clots can form during surgical procedures because a person is lying flat on the operating table without moving. Normally, regular muscular contractions of the legs propel the blood back up through the legs and body to the heart. If a person is simply lying flat and not moving at all for a significant period of time, the blood can stagnate or pool in the veins and a blood clot can form. While this is true of anyone who is still for extensive periods of time, it is more of a problem in the overweight population in whom the added fat further slows the return of venous blood.

Another group of people who are at increased risk above and beyond that of the average overweight population are those people who have a kind of metabolic or genetic clotting disorder. Such disorders can be very subtle and can occasionally remain undiagnosed prior to an operation.

One way surgeons and patients can combat unexpected clotting problems is for an experienced weight-loss center to have a clear-cut repeated policy and mechanisms in place to prevent blood clots. At our center, for example, every patient wears pneumatic sequential compression stockings during operations. These stockings, which look like something out of a science fiction movie, squeeze the legs, ankles and feet and serve to propel the blood up the veins and back to the heart, in close to the same manner normal muscle contractions would. We put the stockings on the patient and start the stockings squeezing before the procedure begins. This results in a dramatic reduction of the risk of blood clotting, even in those patients who have a metabolic or genetic clotting disorder.

The more experienced the surgeon, the better the chances of avoiding blood clots. This is because of the length of time it takes for the procedure. A less-experienced surgeon may take two, three or even four hours performing the LRYGB, for example, An experienced surgeon, who already has a good safety record and has performed hundreds of LRYGB procedures, will typically do the operation in about an hour. It's not a race – speed alone isn't the important thing. It's that the less time the patient spends on the operating table, flat and without normal movement and muscular contractions that move the blood through the veins, the better. So, in the end, performing the surgery quickly, in and of itself, significantly reduces the risk of blood clots.

One more way to reduce the risk of blood clots is to use a low-dose blood thinner, such as heparin or enoxeparin. This kind of medication is often given by injection before or after an operation. Blood-thinning medications reduce the risk of blood clots even further, but they can also elevate the risk of bleeding slightly. As with many challenging decisions regarding the care of surgical patients, the decision to employ a blood-thinning medication requires a careful balancing of the risks of bleeding versus the risks of clotting.

Finally, a last method that can be employed to prevent blood clots involves the placement of a type of filter in the large veins that bring the returning blood from the legs back to the heart, the inferior vena cava. Inferior vena cava filters (also called Greenfield filters) are very successful at preventing blood clots from traveling from the legs to the heart. While they don't prevent blood clots, per se, they do in fact result in a significantly decreased risk for developing serious consequences or complications from blood clots.

Infection

Infection occurs in approximately 1 percent of all surgical incisions regardless of the type of surgery, primarily as a result of gram-positive bacteria that live on skin and throughout the body. Modern antibiotics and preoperative scrubs have dramatically reduced the risks of these types of infections from the days when it was 10 or 20 percent to the standard of perhaps 1 percent.

In most cases, this type of infection isn't a serious complication. It may result in the need for postoperative antibiotics or incising and draining a small abscess at the surgical site, but this is not considered life-threatening, except in very rare cases.

In recent years media attention has focused on some aggressive hospital bacteria that have resulted in serious infections and death. The most common of these is called methicillin-resistant staphylococcus aureus or MRSA. The prevalence of these drug-resistant bacteria has increased in recent years, and infections can be more serious. Some patients are particularly susceptible to staph infections, and they have a history of them occurring in the groin, back or other skin and soft tissues. And obesity is a major risk factor.[70] This is due in part to the impaired blood supply through the extensive subcutaneous fat. The infection-fighting and infection-preventing cells of the body have to travel to the skin to counter these kinds of infections. Obesity makes that process more difficult because the cells have to travel through extensive fat to get to the skin.

We have seen a few such infection cases in our region, but none that required extraordinary treatments to resolve. Some centers and regions of the country have not been so lucky – so it may be worth asking your surgeon if this has been a frequent problem at your hospital or center.

If you have a history of repeated staph infections, you can take steps to avoid another occurring at the time of your weight-loss surgery by doing the following:

» **Inform your surgeon**

» **Consider a preoperative scrub at home with Hibiclens or other antibacterial properties**

» **Lose weight preoperatively**

» **Ask about the prevalence of MRSA at the facility**

However, another type of infection can be considerably more serious. This type occurs internally and results in either peritonitis (inflammation of the thin membrane that lines the abdominal wall and covers most of the organs of the body) or an abscess (a round pocket of fluid with infection) within the abdomen. Such infections are generally caused by microorganisms that escape from the inner lining of the intestine or stomach and travel outside these organs into the peritoneal cavity (the space inside the abdomen where the intestines are). Modern antibiotics and, in some cases, bowel preparations (an oral laxative that reduces the amount of waste, and bacteria, within the intestines the day before surgery) have contributed to the reduction of this type of infection but have not eliminated them.

Types of Procedures, Types of Risks

When you're contemplating an operation, you need to consider the risks. With modern minimally invasive weight-loss procedures, the risks have been reduced considerably as the science has expanded and more and more surgeons have improved expertise. The best understanding of your own risk will come from a discussion between you and your surgeon of your own health status and the specific procedure planned.

Risks with outpatient weight-loss operations are different for each procedure, so each should be considered separately.

LAGB Risks

Short-term complications for the LAGB procedure include infection, bleeding and complications around the site of the port. Longer term complications include band slippage (movement of the band within the body), dyphagia (difficulty swallowing), band erosion and problems of dislodgement or flipping of the access port.

There have been a limited number of cases in which the gastric band has had to be removed. In an extensive series of more than 2,700 bariatric surgeries performed by a single center, the band was removed in 3.7 percent of patients over a period of 10 years, largely because of complications from erosions and slippage.[71-73] This amounts to three to four people out of 100. Most surgeons in this field believe the risks of these types of problems have fallen significantly since this study, due to improvements in the design of the bands and the techniques of the surgeons implanting them.

There are also issues of how tight to make the band. A band could be too tight, producing a sensation of very tight restriction and making it difficult for the patient to drink liquids. A band producing tightness or near complete restriction is a complication that occurs in as many as 1 to 3 percent of procedures. It is a frustrating problem and can take days to resolve as the postoperative swelling goes down. During that time the patient will probably have to remain in a hospital on an IV drip for hydration. While it is not an unusual complication, the odds of experiencing such a complication are considerably reduced by choosing an experienced bariatric surgeon. And a tight band is not regarded as a serious complication, more like an inconvenience, as the patient has to wait around in the hospital for swelling to go down.

Conversion to an open incision could become necessary due to a number of causes, but may occur because of technical difficulties during the procedure or because of excessive bleeding. But again excessive bleeding occurs in less than 1 percent of operations performed by experienced surgeons. If an open incision becomes necessary, then the patient would probably require admission to a hospital.

LRYGB Risks

The laparoscopic RYGB procedure is a technically more complex and advanced procedure than the LAGB and requires a bariatric surgeon with specialized skill and training in that specific procedure. It isn't a procedure that's right for every surgeon to handle in an outpatient setting.

Most of the patients undergoing the laparoscopic RYGB procedure have a hospital stay of between 24 and 40 hours. So, while this book is focused on the changing landscape of weight-loss surgery, which has led to the dramatic revolution from major invasive open procedures to modern minimally invasive outpatient procedures, be aware that the state-of-the-art LRYGB weight-loss surgery for many patients in most states will still require a short hospital stay, and the procedure at most practices is considered *not quite outpatient surgery.*

In the hands of a skilled surgeon, LRYGB can be performed in about an hour, and patients generally can be discharged from the hospital in less than 24 hours. Once a surgeon has performed perhaps 500 to 1,000 of the LRYGB procedures in the hospital setting, it is possible to perform LRYGB in an outpatient setting, in selected patients who don't have excessive health risks or high BMIs.

Outpatient centers usually don't allow patients to stay more than 23 hours, so the patient must be extra motivated to head home within that time frame. Sometimes this motivation stems from a desire to be away from the hospital setting, a desire to return to the comforts of home and the desire to minimize costs. A motivated patient will generally do the preop work and be prepared, having stuck to a meal-replacement diet, lost the preoperative weight and attended classes so as to know what to expect.

Properly prepared, a motivated patient who wants to recover faster and get back home is a good thing. But the sooner you leave the facility, statistically the higher the chance you'll return with complications after some types of weight-loss surgery. A patient who leaves after only five hours might return with nausea and vomiting. The concerns about leaving the surgical facility too quickly need to be weighed against the risks of remaining in the facility, exposed to bacteria and discomfort.

In some geographic areas, regulations allow outpatient surgery centers to permit patients to stays up to 72 hours. So, in such a facility, almost every LRYGB procedure would be considered "outpatient."

In nearly all cases, the gastric bypass procedure can be performed with a laparoscopic or minimally invasive approach. For outpatient LRYGB surgery, we carefully select motivated patients who are low-risk candidates who can be safely discharged home within the 23-hour time window. This is still a difference of hours – not days.

Today, at WBI Center 99 percent of RYGB procedures are performed laparoscopically, making it more likely the patient can be released at less than 23 hours in the surgical facility, and thus making LRYGB an outpatient procedure. However, somewhat inexplicably, there are still surgeons across the country that perform RYGB as an open procedure. Some 25 to 30 percent of RYGB procedures are still done as open operations, with the attendant hospital stay.

According to our data at Western Bariatric Institute, most people who truly want an outpatient procedure choose LAGB or LSG; LRYGB usually requires a one- or two-night hospital stay, though if performed with a laparoscopic procedure and in the morning, it's possible to return home within 23 hours.

I generally counsel my patients that they will stay in the hospital one or two nights and experience recovery times of one to two weeks. Nearly everyone has responsibilities in daily life, from regular jobs to families and kids; because of the nature of the operation I recommend patients plan for two weeks off from these activities before returning full-bore. This allows most people plenty of time to recover and prepare to move forward with their lives.

For most people, this short hospital stay is easily accomplished and reimbursed without financial strain. In fact, in many cases, this rather short hospital stay is unexpectedly welcome news for the insurance companies who were expecting to get hit for a full four-, five-, six- or seven-night hospital stay.

Patient Story: Heather T.

Procedure: **LRYGB**
Weight lost: **127 pounds**

I know that this surgery is not for everyone, but this was the surgery for me! The reason why I wanted the surgery was because I had two small boys, bad health and bad eating habits. My surgeon and his awesome office staff gave me the power to re-invent my life. The very same day I got out of the hospital from having surgery, I started walking. At two weeks, swimming and working out. I don't need plastic surgery; my body is beautiful and healthy. You will always want to take care of yourself because it is so much easier now. Why would you go through such a major surgery and waste it? I needed to learn about what was good for me to eat and drink. Almost two years out, I can eat well, but I learned meals, portions, protein, low carb. This surgery gave me the confidence in so many ways to become what I always wanted to be.

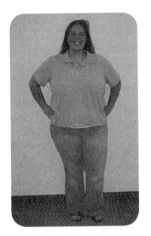

Heather before

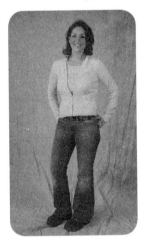

Heather after

Western Bariatric Institute obtains pre-authorization from insurance plans for weight-loss surgery. Sometimes this authorization indicates the number of days expected for hospitalization, and, while we generally have patients in the hospital one to two days, it is not surprising to see authorizations returned for five to six days. The reasons for this often stem from outdated systems used by the insurers, who are using their experience from open abdominal operations to plan the hospital stays.

This "not quite outpatient surgery" in most cities cannot be performed at a truly outpatient weight-loss surgery center, for the majority of cases. In most cases the regulations preclude surgical procedures that require stays longer than 23 hours. Which doesn't mean you shouldn't consider this kind of operation. Every individual's circumstances are different, so every individual should have a frank and open conversation with a skilled and experienced bariatric surgeon and make an individual decision. It may very well be the case where the most appropriate option is a minimally invasive weight-loss procedure that is "not quite outpatient".

For patients undergoing LRYGB at our outpatient facility, I usually keep patients in the facility overnight for observation; the patients are discharged early the next morning. In the rare event that complications arise and hospital admission becomes necessary, there's already a plan in place for the patient to be admitted to the hospital for further evaluation or treatment.

Beyond mortality risk, the main short-term complications for LRYGB procedures stem from potential problems associated with the tissue connection of the stomach pouch to the intestine or between two parts of the intestine. Among the most serious complications, the most common are:

» **Leaking at the anastamosis site**

» **Bleeding**

» **Bowel obstruction**

» **Pulmonary embolus (blood clot in the lungs)**

These potentially life-threatening complications can be corrected by early recognition of the problem and proper intervention. In the case of leaks, serious bleeding or bowel obstruction, surgery is often needed to correct the problem. In the case of a blood clot, medication is given to thin the blood and dissolve the clot.

Complications that can occur later (over weeks to months) include anastamotic stricture (narrowing of the tissue connecting the stomach pouch to the intestine), marginal ulcer (formation of an ulcer or sore on the inside lining of the stomach pouch), vitamin deficiency caused by lack of vitamin supplementation and bowel obstruction. Each of these complications can be corrected by accurate diagnosis and medical treatment, and there's time to sort them out, usually with office visits and tests.

Bleeding

Bleeding is a fairly rare complication occurring in less than 1 percent of weight-loss operations. The literature, across the board, shows that minimally invasive operations have consistently had a lower risk of bleeding than open procedures.

It's not entirely clear why this is the case. It could be the magnification of the camera system on the surgical site during laparoscopy allows a surgeon to stem bleeding where it wouldn't be possible during open procedures. For whatever reason, the risk of bleeding with laparoscopic RYGB is quite low, a portion of 1 percent, meaning there's less than one in 100 chances you'll experience significant bleeding, require a blood transfusion or a return trip to the operating room to correct bleeding if you choose LRYGB and an experienced surgeon.

Bleeding from staple lines after surgery can sometimes occur. Both bleeding during the operation and bleeding from staple lines after surgery are risks more common in people taking blood-thinning medicines such as Coumadin or heparin and its derivatives. In addition, patients who take aspirin, Plavix and ibuprofen, as well as other medications that may affect the aggravation of platelets (an important part of forming a blood clot), may experience elevated risks of postoperative hemorrhage. In most cases, the bleeding will stop on its own without any special treatment other than possibly reversing the effects of an anticoagulant (with additional medication). Generally, bleeding from the staple lines or bleeding from the operation would occur in the hours directly following surgery while the patient was still in the hospital or surgery center. It is possible that slow or steady bleeding could result in light-headedness, pallor and racing heart rate after return home, making a call to the doctor necessary.

Even given how low the odds are, it is still possible a person could end up needing a blood transfusion, an endoscopy (a non-surgical procedure to examine and cauterize an organ using a flexible fiber optic tube passed down the esophagus) or even further surgery to stop excessive or persistent bleeding.

It is always important to tell your surgeon if you have a propensity to bleed more than what is considered normal during surgical procedures (for example, if you have received multiple blood transfusions during routine operations) or if you are taking any medications, especially those that thin the blood. In addition, if you have a personal history of blood clots (called thromboembolism), either in the legs or those that have traveled to the lungs, make sure to tell your surgeon about this so your risks can be better assessed.

Anastomotic Leak

The most important determinant of the risk of intra-abdominal infection is the risk of anastomotic leak. In LRYGB surgery there are two sets of connections (anastamoses) created. The first of these occurs from the small stomach pouch to the Roux limb of the intestine, and the second of these occurs from the Roux limb of the intestine to the rest of the intestinal stream.

Either of these sites of tissue connection can result in a leak, which can be quite dangerous and lead to peritonitis or intra-abdominal abscess. While the risk of these complications is about 1 percent, that does not mean that 1 percent of all patients undergoing gastric bypass surgery will develop peritonitis and serious infection. An experienced and careful bariatric surgeon will have had several if not many leaks occur in patients in the past. The surgeon will know the signs and symptoms of a leak and be able to make the diagnosis of a leak early before serious infection or peritonitis can set in. (*See Appendix E for a discussion on the signs and symptoms of a leak.*)

At Western Bariatric Institute, in the first 1,000 operations the risk of anastamotic leak was approximately 3 percent. In the second 1,000 operations the risk of anastomotic leak was 0.3 percent. In the third 1,000 cases the risk of leak was 0.2 percent. The experience of having performed many hundreds of LRYGB procedures has lead to some important conscious and subconscious learning about the ideal way to form the stomach pouch and the ideal way to form the stomach-intestinal connection.

What we've learned at Western Bariatric Institute is that the critical difference between one operation and the next is caused by the different anatomy of individual patients and the tissue quality of each individual. For us, experience with so many individuals in so many operations has allowed us to adapt to many unexpected findings and anatomies and create healthy, safe, solid, non-leaking anastomoses.

The vast majority of leaks that do happen occur between the stomach pouch and the small intestine. It is much less common for the downstream intestine-to-intestine connection to result in a leak.

Despite the levels of safety attained in today's weight-loss operations, the anastomotic leak remains the most serious complication of the LRYGB procedure and is probably the cause of the majority of deaths reported in the 30 days directly following surgery.

Tissues and Leaks

There's been a great deal of research into the cause of these leaks. During surgery most bariatric surgeons employ a variety of endoscopic stapling techniques to create the anastomosis. In order to create a connection where one hasn't been before, the surgeon must first make incisions to free the tissue that will be moved and then staple or suture the tissue to create the new connection (a procedure also often used to remove a segment of the intestine and re-connect the ends, to treat benign diseases such as polyps, diverticulosis, growths, masses, ulcers or unusual bleeding, and for cancers and lymphoma of the stomach or intestines).

Whether the surgery being performed is for direct treatment of disease or for weight loss, the surgeon is creating connections between two sets of tissues that were not previously connected. And, in general, it is believed that when a leak occurs, it is because the cells of the tissues that have been connected fail to adequately mesh together and form a natural biological connection. (You can picture this basically as a cut on the finger that removes a section of flesh. The two sides of the cut need to be brought together in order to heal. Healing may take longer if the tissues on the two sides don't mesh together to form the missing flesh.)

In order to form the best, strongest possible connection when the tissues are connected to form the anastomosis, certain conditions need to be present. There needs to be a good, healthy supply of blood to the tissues involved, which requires the patient to be healthy and not suffering from anemia or a compromised immune system. There also needs to be an absence of tension at the site where the connection is created – the tissue needs to not be straining to make the connection; a strain can cause a tear and therefore a leak.

These two factors alone are probably the most important issues with any type of gastrointestinal connection, but there are additional factors that can complicate a procedure. Chronic steroid use, a compromised immune system from liver disease, poor nutrition, cancer or severe circulatory problems may affect the adequacy of the blood supply to the tissues, making it difficult for the connection to hold without leaks. Which is to say a young, healthy patient with no problems other than weight would be the ideal candidate for an LRYGB procedure (or any surgical procedure, for that matter). But don't worry; all the studies we cite here, including our own data of more than 3,000 weight-loss operations, involve people of all ages, many with substantial medical problems, just like the medical problems listed above.

A patient is at risk for a leak usually only for the first 24 to 48 hours after surgery. In fact the vast majority of leaks will occur within eight hours of surgery. Very, very rarely, can a leak occur several days after surgery.

Detecting Leaks

The signs and symptoms of a leak vary between individuals, but most often involve rapid heart rate, then rapid breathing, fever and increased pain. The first thing a surgeon does when it is believed a leak has occurred is immediately confirm the diagnosis and act to repair it.

Some surgeons use imaging studies, such as an upper gastrointestinal contrast study or CT scan (the traditional CAT scan we've all heard of) to determine if a leak has in fact occurred. Such tests aren't perfect but can help a surgeon pinpoint trouble. Often if it is believed a patient's anastomosis has developed a leak, the surgeon will return the patient to the operating room for a re-exploration, either laparoscopically or, at this point, through an open abdominal incision. In my own practice the test employed depends on the level of likelihood that there may be a leak. As with other experienced surgeons in this field, we at Western Bariatric Institute have tried all of the above tests and procedures. We've even performed exploratory open surgery and discovered patients who didn't have leaks at all but rather some other processes mimicking symptoms of leaks. (For example, a patient with extreme anxiety reported abnormally high levels of pain and elevated heart rate. What seemed a very high possibility of a leak proved to be a healthy, normal anastamosis at laparoscopy.)

An Ounce of Prevention

One of the ways we've found to protect against the possibility of anastomotic leaks at Western Bariatric Institute has been to perform a pressure test of the gastrojejunal anastomosis while the patient is still in the operating room. We test the tenacity of the pouch before ending the operation. So, once the operation is finished, and we're sure the results are excellent, and there's little chance of leaks, we test the anastomosis. We pass a soft tube down the esophagus to the point of the anastomosis, prevent intestinal outflow from the anastomosis, and fill the stomach pouch with a blue-dyed saline. This puts pressure on the stomach pouch and on the new connection and allows us to make certain there are no leaks. If there are, we can make repairs, revisions or reinforcements right then and there, making sure we've got a tight seal with no chance of leaks.

Now that we've done some 1,500 leak tests, it's become increasingly uncommon for us to find any leaks during the operation. I'd estimate we find subtle leakage in one out of every 100 cases. Even then it's not certain those cases would have lead to clinical leak and infection, but testing for leaks during the actual operation gives us an extra edge in achieving a high degree of safety and security.

A leak that is detected early usually creates no long-term complications or consequences, but when a leak isn't discovered promptly it can result in severe complications.

Whatever test is used to check for a leak, usually the follow-up treatment by a savvy team of surgeons and nurses that employs early and aggressive detection and intervention will successfully mitigate the consequences of a leak.

LSG Risks

Laparoscopic sleeve gastrectomy (LSG) involves removing a significant portion of the stomach, permanently reducing the size of the stomach overall. The level of invasiveness and complexity is in between that of the LAGB (less invasive/complex) and the LRYGB (more invasive/complex). Because of this, the mortality risk is quite low, on par with the figures cited above.[74-77]

As with the LAGB and the LRYGB, LSG involves a laparoscopic procedure on the stomach with general anesthesia. Because general anesthesia is involved, there are some risks to be considered. The procedure can be performed in the outpatient setting, often with discharge within the 23-hour window. The chief complications seen with LSG are:

» **Vomiting**

» **Leaking at the cut edge of the stomach**

» **Bleeding**

» **Conversion to open procedure**

In LSG, part of the stomach is removed, leaving the remaining stomach smaller, narrower and more tube-like.

The result is a form of restriction of the stomach and on how much the patient can eat. Sometimes in the immediate postoperative period, the surgery can result in nausea and vomiting that can take days to resolve. Usually, with preparation, antinausea medications and a liquid diet, patients can avoid this and still go home after the overnight stay, but not always. Occasionally patients need to stay in the hospital for intravenous hydration and wait until the swelling goes down and the newly reduced stomach settles down before going home.

LSG doesn't involve an anastamosis, but it does involve a long staple line along the edge of the newly-shrunken stomach. So, while it is quite rare, a leak could potentially occur anywhere along the edge of the stomach where it was cut and stapled or sutured. The detection and consequences would be the same as those discussed above for leaks after LRYGB operations.

Other complications, such as conversion to open surgery and bleeding, can occur in rare cases. Overall the risks of developing problems after an LSG procedure appear to fall in between those of the LAGB and the LRYGB and are rare overall.

What we don't know is whether more patients with LSG will, over the long term, develop some nutritional abnormalities or problems with gastroesophageal reflux (heartburn). And perhaps the most important thing we don't know is whether or not, over the long term, the LSG will remain durable and not lead to stretching out of the stomach pouch or tube. Based on what I know about LRYGB and other types of surgery, it seems likely to me that some people will develop dilation of the new stomach tube over time, but whether this will occur in many of the patients undergoing this procedure or only a few, only time will tell.

Risks of not Undergoing Surgical Weight Loss

The risks of weight-loss operations must be held up and compared to the risks of not having a surgical weight-loss procedure. Consider the risks faced by the decision not to undergo a modern weight-loss operation and choosing instead to either work through a nonsurgical weight-loss program (there are several excellent programs, as well as other not-so-excellent programs) or to simply ignore the whole problem of being overweight.

Several studies have shown that the risks of not undergoing weight-loss operations for the seriously overweight are substantial.[61] Studies that provide a nonsurgical control group of overweight patients indicate a much greater risk of heart disease, diabetes and mortality over the years following the studies compared to those patients who underwent weight-loss surgery.

A study that compared the surgical group to a group of seriously overweight people undergoing an extensive medically supervised (nonsurgical) weight-loss program (something very few people actually do), found the medical group fared far worse in terms of weight loss and health outcomes.[37] This is not to say you should not enroll in a high quality nonsurgical, medically-supervised weight-loss program. In fact, it may be the best first step you can take if you are serious about losing the weight.

Many people, especially those with a lower BMI (say, less than 30) can enjoy great success with a medically-supervised weight-loss program that employs counseling, dietary coaching, meal replacements, exercise, prescription drugs and consultation with doctors and psychologists. However, it's difficult to find programs that can combine all these elements, along with support groups and motivational challenges for patients, under one roof.

Most health insurance plans won't pay for medically supervised nonsurgical weight-loss programs. In addition, people with BMIS of more than 30 have a harder time achieving their weight-loss and health goals without operations.

The bottom line is that with or without surgery, losing the weight and keeping it off requires commitment, support and the right tools. The ideal approach may be integrating both surgery and a great medically supervised plan into your long-term approach to lose the weight, keep it off and stay healthy. The key is to understand that every month of living with the extra weight incurs risks, so calculate those carefully into your analysis of the risks of outpatient weight-loss surgery.

Considering that weight gain is the primary risk factor for elevations of cholesterol and lipids, high blood pressure, diabetes, heart disease and shortened life expectancy, it stands to reason that the risks of not aggressively bringing the weight down are pretty substantial.

Always bear in
mind that your own
resolution to succeed
is more important
than any other one
thing.

– ABRAHAM LINCOLN

Food for Thought

» Today's minimally invasive weight-loss operations are significant and life-changing, and a body of data shows that for patients with a BMI of more than 35, <u>not</u> undergoing a surgical weight-loss procedure is more risky than doing so.

» The 1991 National Institutes of Health Consensus Conference statement on obesity addressed the topic of weight-loss procedures. At the time, the mortality rate for the open procedures exceeded 5 percent. Despite this, the statement indicated that the risks of remaining seriously overweight exceeded the risks of having the operations.

» Many weight-loss procedures performed today are the same in theory as they were in the 1980s and 90s but modifications have enhanced their effectiveness while drastically cutting the risks.

» The best way to minimize any risks associated with undergoing bariatric or weight-loss surgery is to seek out an experienced, well-trained surgeon with a proven track record.

» Surgeons who have performed 20 procedures operate with a 6 percent mortality risk. Surgeons who have performed more than 250 procedures operate with a virtually 0 percent risk.

» Without surgery, losing the weight and keeping it off requires commitment, support and the right tools. For some people a medically supervised program combining counseling, dietary coaching, meal replacements, exercise, prescription drugs and consultation with doctors and psychologists can help, but finding a program with all the right components can be challenging.

» Weight gain is the primary risk factor for elevations of cholesterol and lipids, high blood pressure, diabetes, heart disease and shortened life expectancy. The risks for not aggressively bringing down the weight are substantial.

I know the price of success: dedication, hard work, and an unremitting

devotion to the things you want to see happen.

– FRANK LLOYD WRIGHT

4

Choice

TODAY'S SURGICAL WEIGHT-LOSS procedures offer a variety of choices. If you decide to undergo a weight-loss operation, many of the choices will be up to you. There are choices in procedure and choices in what experienced, well-trained bariatric surgeon you choose to perform your procedure. You'll need to choose which outpatient surgery center to use or which hospital if you choose to have the operation performed in a traditional hospital setting.

Every choice is important when it comes to your health and well-being, and before making any decisions you should research your options as thoroughly as possible and understand the pros and cons of each choice. Reading this book is a great start, but don't stop here! (*See Appendix C for more sources of information.*)

Choosing a Bariatric Surgeon

When you've made the decision to move ahead with a weight-loss operation, either LAGB, LRYGB, LSG or perhaps a different procedure, it is time to select the right program and the right surgeon.

You can start your research with one of the specialty societies for weight-loss surgery: the American College of Surgeons (ACS) or the American Society of Metabolic and Bariatric Surgery (ASMBS). The effort these organizations have put forward over the last several years to identify the Centers of Excellence around the country is one that really should be commended. The centers you can find at the ACS site (*www.FACS.org*) or the ASMBS site (*www.ASBS.org*) are good places to start in selecting the right program and the right surgeon. However, there are many excellent centers and surgeons outside the Centers of Excellence classification system.

It's always important to talk to as many people and get as many recommendations as possible from people both within the health care industry and without. Talk to everyone you can and try to gain as much information as possible about the surgeon and the program. And then compare. Talk to people involved with competing programs and centers, go online and take a look at the various programs available. You can use the one I work with as a reference (*www.WesternBariatricInstitute.com*), and there are many other excellent programs around the country that you can start to get a sense of by looking online.

The Web is one place where people have given lots of feedback about various programs, and it's easy to access this information (*Appendix C should help*). By reading through the comments from past and present patients, you may gain further insight. You might also check out my blog and read comments, or leave one yourself (*www.SasseGuide.com*).

Not every piece of the puzzle that you find will create a full picture in and of itself, but each will give you a little bit more information and help you feel a little bit more comfortable about your decision.

Choosing an Outpatient Surgery Center

When it comes to choosing the facility at which you will undergo a weight-loss operation, you have many choices. You may have an established relationship with a hospital in your community. Your insurance plan might have a list of contracted facilities that are approved for "in network" reimbursement, and these facilities may include hospitals and outpatient surgery centers. Your surgeon may also have a relationship with a specific outpatient surgery center. One of your considerations will be whether or not to investigate and choose any of these different options.

What should you look for?

Your top consideration should be that the center provides a safe, comfortable and professional environment for your surgical experience. Some people find the hospital environment too clinical or sterile and cold. Others feel more comfortable in the larger, standard hospital environment.

Some people may prefer the security of knowing that a full hospital apparatus is available should any problems arise and that an intensive care unit and complex radiology department are available if there are complications following surgery. However, since all outpatient surgery centers have contingency plans in case complications arise, and since many are associated or even physically attached to major hospitals, more and more patients are comfortable with outpatient surgery centers. And for the most part, other hospital features won't be necessary for the vast majority of patients undergoing minimally invasive weight-loss surgery.

You should also factor in the convenience of scheduling at an outpatient surgical center, which is easier than scheduling through a hospital. This means you have more options for scheduling the time and date of your operation, which may make it easier for friends and family to arrange your transport to and from the center and your care after you return home.

No Quick Fix

One thing that every bariatric expert can agree on is that weight-loss operations, whether for adolescents or anyone else, are not quick fixes. Success after weight-loss surgery comes to those who commit – mind, body and soul – to long-term behavior change, exercise and good food choices. It is hard work. For many people, weight-loss operations change nearly impossible battles into very winnable battles. But no matter what media coverage depicts weight-loss surgery as an easy fix, it most certainly is not. Adolescents and adults must take advantage of every bit of the counseling available and utilize support groups and establish long-term, positive habits for success.

Last, you'll want to visit the facility and see the kind of environment provided and determine whether it provides a comfort level that is acceptable to you. Many outpatient surgery centers make an effort to provide a warm and pleasant experience for both patient and visitors, who may be spending time in the waiting room.

Making a choice of where to have surgery may seem intimidating, but really you're making the decision the same way you make other important decisions in your life – by gathering the facts and comparing your options. I suggest you start with the surgeon you're interviewing for your weight-loss surgery. Ask where the surgeon prefers to perform procedures and then go and visit the facilities. You can learn a great deal by walking through a facility or asking for a tour. You can gain a sense of the professionalism of the center and gauge the cleanliness with your own eyes. Ask the surgeon why he or she prefers one center over another. Ask the surgeon how many weight-loss surgical procedures have been performed at the facility.

When interviewing the surgeon, here's a list of questions you can start with:

1. How many weight-loss procedures has the surgeon performed?

2. How many of them were performed in an outpatient center or outpatient setting?

3. Which procedures does the surgeon perform?

4. Is the surgeon a Board-Certified surgeon, a Fellow of the American College of Surgeons?

5. Is the surgeon a member of the American Society of Metabolic and Bariatric Surgery?

6. How many years has the surgeon been performing bariatric surgery?

7. What preoperative diet and weight-loss strategies are recommended? (*See Chapter 5 for more information about what sort of preoperative diets are standard.*)

8. What postoperative education and support is provided?

9. How often do support groups meet? (*See Chapter 5 for more information on support groups.*)

10. What testing and preoperative evaluation (*see Chapter 5 for more information*) does the surgeon require?

A lot of surgeons and centers make all this type of information available on their Web sites and in patient materials. You may be able to obtain all the facts without taking up all your time with the surgeon focusing on these topics. Instead you may want to spend some of that time talking about *you*, about the uniqueness of your case, and how the surgeon feels he or she can best help you achieve your goals.

Adolescents and Outpatient Weight-Loss Surgery

Adolescents and children present a particularly challenging subgroup for health care providers, surgeons, parents and families. As surgeons, we want to help, but we are also aware of the complexity of obesity as a disease and its relationship to both the developing psyche and body of a child or adolescent. There has been a good deal of research directed at the topic of weight-loss surgery for adolescents, and the topic remains controversial.[78-81]

On the one hand, people who emphasize the psychosocial aspects of weight gain and unhealthy habits, decision-making and behavioral aspects of this problem point out that children and adolescents have developing brains and have a greater likelihood of changing their lives and resolving weight problems without resorting to surgical procedures. On the other hand, advocates for overweight adolescents point out that it can be considered cruel to withhold valuable treatment for such a devastating prob-lem. They emphasize that the important years of adolescence – high school and college years – are critical for the formation of healthy relationships, self-esteem and career paths and that these formative years set the compass for the direction of these young people's lives.

Adolescent Success

I have performed LAGB surgery on a number of adolescents with strong support of their parents, pediatricians and psychologists. In each case, these adolescents had tried everything to lose weight and understood the seriousness of their decisions. One young man whose parents were both severely overweight felt that he had no chance of attaining a healthy weight in high school without help. Following the LAGB proce-dure he lost 70 pounds and has moved into his senior year with a much healthier body and much healthier self-image.

It is also important to note that the entire recovery process for the out-patient procedure takes about a week. For the young man in question, he was able to have the operation during a break from school and not have to face probing questions about taking a medical leave. The LAGB option allowed him and his family to keep the decision private.

Adolescent weight-loss surgery will probably continue to be a debated topic for years to come, but I think the most important consideration must be the health of the adolescent. In unusual cases where a young person is developing high blood pressure, liver disease and takes insulin for diabetes, we are talking about life-threatening conditions. For other adolescents, the problem of obesity is intertwined with social, behavioral and mood problems and a terrible lack of knowledge about nutrition and health.

Physically, adolescents are usually excellent surgical candidates for medical procedures because they tend to be healthier by virtue of being young. They have not had all the extra years to carry around or develop all the extra weight and generally have not developed conditions such as diabetes and heart disease.

The decision for a weight-loss procedure extends beyond cosmetic considerations. With adolescents, a weight-loss operation is often proactive – a procedure meant to pre-empt the deleterious physical effects of being overweight that will most likely develop as the child enters adulthood.

Our own approach at Western Bariatric Institute has been to perform LAGB surgery for adolescents under the auspices of a research study protocol.[82] It requires that adolescents be seen, evaluated and approved by a psychologist and pediatrician, as well as a parent, prior to entering the program. Only the LAGB is offered, because our surgeons feel the fact that the procedure can be reversed is important when the decision for surgery is made for a minor.

In the past when the only surgical options available were more invasive and more permanent procedures such as biliopancreatic diversion and gastric bypass, it made less sense to offer weight-loss surgery to a wide population of overweight adolescents. There would almost definitely be complications to answer for, and the permanence of the surgical intervention could certainly be questioned by those who point out that minors do not have the same level of decision-making capability as adults.

Some opponents of adolescent weight-loss surgery would also contend that successful weight-loss surgery requires a high level of commitment on the part of the patient. And since adolescents often lack the experience and maturity to make such a deep commitment to lifestyle changes and healthier habits, they should be made to wait a few years until they reach adulthood.

Because the LAGB procedure has a track record of success, a compelling case can be made to make it more available to adolescents. Just as for adults, LAGB surgery is minimally invasive, requiring only a 30- to 40-minute procedure, and is reversible with another fairly minimal procedure and few adverse consequences. There are currently no standard criteria for selecting adolescents for weight-loss surgery. Most centers that perform adolescent weight-loss surgery will consider candidates with a BMI of 35 or greater, as long as the parent and the child are committed to long-term success, and the patient passes the psychological screening.

Aging Individuals and Outpatient Weight-Loss Procedures

Strikingly few seriously overweight individuals live late into life. The medical and health implications and consequences are simply too much as we age. But there are a large number of individuals in their 50s, 60s and 70s who are moderately overweight but lack the tools to successfully lose weight and regain a more active lifestyle. These individuals are at high risk for serious health problems and early death.

We don't hear as often about the potential benefits of minimally invasive weight-loss procedures for people in their 60s and older, but not only are the benefits considerable, the procedures are now available as outpatient operations for older patients who might not previously have been surgical candidates.

All three procedures discussed – the LAGB, LRYGB and LSG – are usually tolerated well by older patients, and surgeons often choose to work with these patients in the outpatient setting. Many of us working in the field have observed that seniors often tolerate the discomfort and inconvenience of weight-loss procedures and anesthesia with greater aplomb and less pain and suffering than their younger counterparts.

Reversibility is not as crucial a concern in this population as it is with adolescents, but the minimal invasiveness of the procedure is critical. It allows older patients with potentially serious health problems to undergo weight-loss procedures that can move them light years closer to solving problems caused by being overweight.

I must admit that I personally measure success in terms of the contributions an individual makes to her or his fellow human beings.

– MARGARET MEAD

Studies have demonstrated that older patients do well after LAGB and LRYGB surgery and lose weight (though weight loss may be harder for them to achieve with the same magnitude of dramatic results than it is for middle-aged and younger patients).[83-86] My colleagues and I know that the odds of making the needed changes at this stage of life without surgical intervention are often very slim indeed. I have performed LAGB and LRYGB surgery on a number of patients in their 60s and 70s and have been pleased to watch them prove they can make good use of their new weapons in the weight-loss war. These patients have been able to lose weight, improve their health, increase their activities and elevate their quality of life.

Unfortunate Financial Realities

Seniors face an additional battle in weight loss: that of getting their weight-loss procedures covered by insurance. Although more and more conventional insurance plans are covering weight-loss operations, and so is Medicare, that doesn't mean seniors are going to have financial access to surgical procedures. Once a person turns 65 and becomes automatically covered under Medicare, most surgeons will not accept that patient as a candidate for weight-loss surgery.

Why not? Because insurance companies don't seem to understand that a successful weight-loss operation takes more than a scalpel and some anesthesia. Medicare "covers" the service and pays the facility and the surgeon at a rate insufficient to cover costs for the surgical practice to perform the procedure, let alone provide education and follow-up to the patient – important components to successful surgical weight-loss programs.

As a result, most practices quickly close their doors to patients on Medicare. Our own practice was, until recently, the only Center of Excellence program west of the Mississippi River to accept new Medicare patients, and now even we have had to limit the number of these cases each year, performed as a type of community service.

The problem is compounded by the fact that surgeons, by virtue of being "Medicare providers," are not allowed to accept fees other than the standard Medicare fee schedule for covered benefits including bariatric surgery. What that means is simply this: Even if a senior wants to pay cash in order to undergo minimally invasive weight-loss surgery, surgeons, being Medicare providers, can't accept it. In the last couple years, my office has been inundated by frustrated seniors who would clearly benefit from weight-loss procedures and have offered sizeable sums of cash to have someone in my practice perform the operations. But since all of the surgeons in the practice are Medicare providers, we are legally prevented from providing this service.

I wish I knew what's going to happen in the future as our population ages and the number of overweight individuals age 65 and older grows. I suspect one of three things will occur that will allow minimally invasive weight-loss procedures to become more available for more seniors:

1. Medicare will raise its rates to a level that allows surgeons to provide the service without paying money out of their own pockets (not the most likely option).

2. Many more general surgeons offering weight-loss surgery will accept Medicare patients as they are growing their practices and refining their skills.

3. An increasing number of surgeons will drop their status as Medi-

care providers in order to accept patients outside the Medicare program. But while this will open the door for some seniors, it isn't the solution for the greater number of seniors who still won't be able to pay for the procedures independently.

Insurance and Finances

One of the reasons outpatient weight-loss surgery is growing quickly in popularity is that outpatient procedures are much less expensive than the inpatient procedures performed in the early days. And more and more patients are paying out-of-pocket.[87]

As weight-loss surgery has become increasingly recognized as safe and effective and no longer a mysterious, time-consuming and expensive open procedure, the demand has grown. Many more insurance carriers now cover weight-loss surgical procedures than did just a few years ago, but there are some insurance carriers that either don't cover the procedures or make it very difficult to get coverage. Some carriers place onerous obstacles and high hurdles in front of patients who want to undergo weight-loss procedures. Many try to make it so difficult that patients will give up their quests.

Rather than giving up, many patients are opting to pay out-of-pocket. The decision has advantages and disadvantages, putting the patient in charge of many of his or her own health care

Insurance Frustration

One of the most frustrating things in the world for me, and my patients, is to grapple with Medicare and other insurance systems that make it hard for people to have access to the health care they need. The costs to run a practice have escalated enormously, mainly in response to these very bureaucracies. Almost every doctor, and especially every surgeon, performs a great deal of middle-of-the-night charity care for indigent patients in need of emergency care. But we limit the amount of elective procedures we will perform without fair reimbursement.

With weight-loss surgery now proven to be so effective in extending life and improving health, the fairest system would be for it to be a covered benefit at a fair rate, just like every other proven medical treatment. That way as providers we could focus on doing the job we love to do: helping people live healthier and longer lives. Instead, some insurers won't cover weight-loss operations at all (making them available to only those who can afford to pay), some cover them fairly and Medicare "covers" them but pays the surgeons less than it costs to provide the services. I know this is frustrating for seniors, and it is frustrating for providers, too.

Certainly this problem is just a microcosm of the whole health care system. I recently learned that almost none of the primary care physicians in my community will accept new Medicare patients, because they cannot afford to accept the low rates. It's even a shock to *my* parents who need a regular doctor today, and what about the baby boomers that will all need primary care doctors tomorrow?

decisions. But one definite effect paying out-of-pocket has is this: patients become highly cost-conscious consumers. And outpatient surgery centers are an economical option for safe and effective weight-loss surgery.

In my market, the Northern Nevada and Lake Tahoe region, in 2001, approximately 2 percent of the patients undergoing weight-loss operations paid cash. In 2007, approximately 8 percent of the patients were cash-paying patients. In many other markets, the percentage of patients paying out-of-pocket is dramatically higher.

For example, cost-conscious patients in the Northern Nevada region would find the outpatient surgery center price substantially lower than having a weight-loss procedure in an area hospital. An LAGB procedure at one of our hospitals, including all personnel and services (such as surgeons, hospital facility fee, anesthesiologists, assistants and equipment) would typically run $25,000 to $28,000. At an outpatient surgery center, the costs drop dramatically to approximately $18,000, including all of the costs listed above, plus extensive classes, nutritional counseling and preoperative education.

With more than 300,000 bariatric surgical procedures expected to be performed annually by 2012, and an increasing percentage of these being paid for exclusively by patients, there will inevitably be a greater demand for outpatient weight-loss surgery. If the cost differences between hospital and outpatient surgery centers remain as they do today, then most patients will continue to choose outpatient surgery centers for their procedures.

Paying Cash for Weight-Loss Procedures: Concerns and Considerations

With an increasing number of people paying for their own weight-loss operations when their insurance carriers won't, important questions and concerns are being raised. For example, what happens if complications arise and more surgery is required? What happens if after surgery the patient needs to be admitted to the hospital for ongoing care? And what happens if there is a complication down the road? Will an insurance company eventually cover these contingencies, or will the patient be exposed to future costs not initially budgeted for?

Solutions for these problems have been found at experienced centers like WBI. But these questions have yet to be widely addressed within the current insurance environment. At this writing, many centers are embarking on programs to create insurance products or warranty products that will allow coverage for many, if not most, complications. Keep in mind that complications in weight-loss surgery are rare in the hands of an experienced bariatric surgeon. So, the discussion pertains to a small percentage of the overall population undergoing weight-loss procedures. Nevertheless, even if we are talking about 1 percent of a group of 300,000 people we are still discussing 3,000 people a year who may experience significant financial concerns if complications arise.

Many centers are developing mechanisms by which additional surgical and hospital services may be covered with the initial costs of the weight-loss procedures. In some cases, these added coverages or benefits do add significantly to the costs of the procedure – anywhere from a few hundred dollars to upward of $1,500 per case. However, by paying the additional coverage, serious financial risks can be avoided.[88]

When making your decisions on a weight-loss procedure, ask your surgeon and your outpatient surgery center staff if they offer such plans or even a less formal means of providing care and coverage should a complication occur. At many centers where there is yet no formal insurance or warranty-type coverage policy in place, agreements are in place to allow for a return to surgery in order to correct complications. Procedures in that event are provided for by the center and the surgeon at little additional cost to the patient. In some cases complications are taken care of at a cost to the patient that covers the expenses and equipment usage for such complications. (But even these "minimum" charges can run in the thousands or tens of thousands if major complications occur.)

Patient Story: Doug T.

Procedure: **LAGB**
Weight lost: **75 pounds**

Prior to surgery, I had been on every diet known to man, adding weight each time. I came off each diet to a blimp size of 274.5 pounds – ouch! I was convinced the only way to lose the weight and keep it off was with surgery. I wanted the bypass, but my doctor convinced me that at my age (66 at the time), I was better for LAGB. Since I have had the LAGB, I agree with him 100 percent. Before my surgery, at 274.5 pounds, I was a slug, sat around and did nothing. Now I play with my grandchildren and build things in my shop. I feel like I am 30 years younger! This has given me a new lease on life. Now at age 67, I feel like I'm 37 after losing all this weight. You have no idea how it feels to be able to go and do things again.

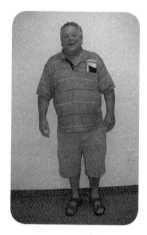

Doug before

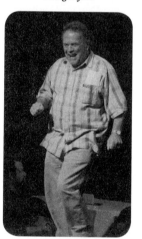

Doug after

This was the type of agreement Western Bariatric had reached in Reno with the inpatient and outpatient surgery centers prior to ever undertaking surgical weight-loss procedures. Now we provide a separate and formalized insurance or warranty policy for each and every patient paying cash for his or her weight-loss operation.

If you are considering a surgical outpatient weight-loss procedure and a formal coverage policy is offered, take it. I can't emphasize enough how valuable it will be to have coverage in place should a complication occur. The extra costs will be well-spent. At WBI, we now offer a coverage policy for most major complications for any patient undergoing weight-loss surgery and paying without help from insurance. Through the BLIS, Inc. program, a premium is added to the overall fees, which covers the cost of additional procedures and hospitalization if such become necessary due to complications arising after surgery.

So, like all forms of insurance, in which we pay a small premium in exchange for coverage of a major potential expense (think of a car insurance policy), this concept involves pooling of risks across a large group of people. The funds from every premium go to pay for that rare case that involves an expensive complication.

Some centers require the extra coverage or policy, and the costs are automatically rolled into the fee charged. This is probably the best way to go. If it's the policy at the center you choose, it's there for your protection. The journey to successful weight loss and long-term health has plenty of challenges without adding the stress of potential financial hardship.

What to Tell (or Not to Tell) Your Boss and Friends

What you choose to tell those around you is your business.

Whether you wish to tell everyone that you are undergoing a surgical weight-loss procedure and enlist their help and support during your journey or whether you wish to maintain absolute privacy about this decision is up to you.

Years ago the logistics of weight-loss surgery required a substantial operation followed by a significant seven- to 10-day hospital stay and lengthy recovery that could last months after the patient returned home. Obviously if the person were missing from work or school for such a long period people were bound to notice and inquire. So, while not impossible, it was certainly improbable to expect a person would be able to maintain complete privacy about the operation.

In addition, before the modern, minimally invasive techniques, candidates for weight-loss surgery tended to be more seriously overweight. Because weight-loss surgery is a risk/benefit decision and in earlier years the risks were greater, it made sense to apply treatment selectively to those candidates who stood to gain greater benefits because their health problems were more severe. Since the results were more dramatic in those cases, results were much more likely to be noticed, as well.

Today things are different. Weight-loss procedures may only result in as little as a one-day absence from work or school. With such a short time away, there's a much better chance of keeping the decision to oneself.

Is secrecy the best course of action for you? That's a discussion to have with your surgeon and your spouse or best support person. And every answer will be individual. I will tell you that it is an important decision you need to make while planning your weight-loss operation, and you need to make it early in the process and share it with your surgeon and surgery center personnel so those involved can take steps to protect your privacy. There is no way to absolutely guarantee privacy, but there are numerous steps that can be taken by the surgeon, surgical staff and surgery center personnel that will markedly reduce the odds of third parties learning of your decision to undergo a weight-loss procedure.

Benefits of Remaining Open About Your Choice

There are benefits to not keeping your decision a secret. For one thing, you can avoid the necessity of lying and any awkward moments secrecy can cause. Keeping the weight-loss operation a secret is bound to lead to some of those awkward moments. The most common and nicest of these is when your friends, neighbors and co-workers begin to ask you what you're doing to lose so much weight. If you are planning to maintain secrecy about the operation, you will need to have an answer ready that you're comfortable using and can use consistently.

If you choose to keep your secret, try out your answer before you're ever put in the position of needing to use it. You may want to indicate you're in a medically supervised weight-loss program and exercising more while eating better. This answer has the advantage of being largely true while somewhat vague. But be prepared for people asking for many more concrete details at that point.

After trying this for a while, even in private, you may decide you are simply more comfortable telling people you had a weight-loss operation and are working very hard at medically supervised weight loss and exercise. Many people will respond positively to this. Those who have struggled with being overweight themselves will respect you for having the courage to do what they couldn't. Some will be jealous. And most will be happy for you. Almost all of them will have many more questions about your surgery, your surgeon and your decision to have the procedure, and usually these questions will reflect admiration for your decisions.

Occasionally you will encounter very ignorant attitudes and people who feel you took the "easy way out." It's up to you whether to try and dissuade them of this misapprehension or leave them to their own beliefs. If you choose to try and explain to them, you might want to mention:

1. It takes hard work, commitment to a program of learning, changing behavior, exercising and adhering to the medically prescribed nutrition and exercise regimen.

2. While the surgery only takes an hour, the process of getting from the decision to have weight-loss surgery to the procedure itself takes a lot of time and effort and classes and evaluations.

3. It made no sense NOT to have the operation, given the health statistics with surgery vs. without surgery.

But mostly you will encounter a community of people who admire you for doing it, who support you and recognize your journey is a difficult one and one that required a great deal of courage and perseverance. Which leads to another reason you might want to consider telling people about your choice: positive effects of having an open support group.

There are numerous studies that describe the benefits of successful long-term weight loss, and most of them point to personal group support as being key. Having a support person or a support group is helpful for long-term challenging behavior modifications of many types, such as stopping smoking or quitting drinking. The National Weight-Loss Registry data points out the importance of support groups for their database of long-term successful weight loss, and weight-loss programs such as WeightWatchers® have long relied on the positive support of group dynamics to further the goals of health and weight loss.

Don't underestimate the value of a support group, especially an organic group comprised of people you see in your everyday life. In addition, your surgeon may recommend or require you to attend a support group either before or after your procedure, or possibly both. These groups provide a forum for people who have had the same types of operations with the same surgical group to support and encourage each other on the weight-loss journey. If your focus is on privacy, it may not be possible for you to take advantage of this component of long-term weight loss.

One more consideration: If you choose to be open about your decision, you may be able to help other people. It is estimated that only around 1 percent of those people who could most benefit from weight-loss operations and enjoy longer, healthier lives ever actually undergo much-needed weight-loss procedures. Many fail to seek effective treatment for their health because they are stymied by concerns about how the procedure is perceived, lack of knowledge about the minimally invasive approach, fear of complications and the judgment of others who don't understand modern weight-loss procedures.

Your openness can help these people learn more about modern weight-loss procedures and other state-of-the-art medical procedures that could help improve the quality and length of their lives. Many patients tell me they only sought weight-loss operations after close friends led the way and then shared the experience, dispelling misconceptions, banishing fears that had prevented them from moving forward with much needed medical intervention. You really can help make a difference, and it may turn out to be one of the most surprisingly rewarding aspects of your own weight-loss journey.

Advantages to Keeping your Decision Private

There may also be some advantages to keeping your decision entirely private. For one thing, people around you may not always approve of or understand your decision to undergo a weight-loss procedure. Most of the time people react quite favorably and quite supportively, but not always. Sharing your decision to undergo a weight-loss operation means exposing yourself to the judgments of others, and this can be uncomfortable if someone in your circle lacks the knowledge and sophistication to appreciate why your decision benefits your health and longevity. I have heard a few stories over the years of patients whose bosses, mothers or siblings forever blamed the weight-loss operation for any health or physical problem that arose. One of my patients, who in the course of a year had sniffles, a sinus infection and a broken leg, found his sister erroneously blaming each of these events on a weight-loss procedure that had occurred four years earlier!

Sharing openly your decision to have a weight-loss procedure may help battle the ignorance of people around you with regard to weight-loss operations, but it just might not be a battle you want to fight.

Another fact to consider when weighing whether or not to share your decision openly is that you just don't have to. Just as you might keep close counsel with respect to any other health problems you have experienced, you may wish to maintain the same level of privacy with respect to this decision. In the end, no matter what your boss, friends or family think or don't think, it is really none of their business.

So, in summary, as I see it, you have three options:

1. The first option is to keep your weight-loss procedure decision a secret. This may spare you from some of the ignorant opinions of others and limit the topic as a conversation item.

2. Be fully open and share your decision with those around you. This may provide some advantages of extra support and encouragement and may help others learn that they too could benefit.

3. Be discreet but honest. I have seen a few people choose this middle ground. I have performed surgery on a number of famous people

who ultimately chose this approach. They wished to minimize the publicity surrounding their decision to undergo weight-loss surgery, and yet they wanted to be open with their immediate family and closest friends. They did attend limited support groups and, if asked, shared that they had indeed undergone weight-loss surgery. But they chose not to mention it unless asked directly about it. And in some cases they took measures to increase the discretion of the practice and the surgery center to decrease the sphere of people who learned of their decision.

Privacy

Your surgeon and his or her practice can help you maintain your privacy. Here are some of the ways:

HIPPA. The privacy compliance law known commonly as HIPAA – Health Insurance Portability and Accountability Act of 1996 – works in your favor if you choose to maintain your privacy about a weight-loss procedure. Your surgeon and your surgeon's staff are required to adhere to HIPAA. Among the many provisions of this law is the strict requirement that practice or center staff not reveal any of your private information, or even that you were a patient, with anyone that you have not authorized.

I should mention that HIPAA does nothing to protect your information from the people who can really do you some harm, namely the insurance industry, the government and law enforcement entities at all levels who request access to your private information. But should a co-worker, a friend, a relative or a journalist call the office to inquire about your status, no information would be given without your prior authorization. I can't resist adding that such privacy concerns have long been a principle of medical care, and HIPAA codified the idea into a cumbersome law that involves an awful lot of trees felled to comply with the paperwork. Hopefully now the noble ethics of the medical field combined with the law work together to prevent abuses of disclosure of information.

Mary

A couple of years ago, I had a patient I'll call "Mary." She came to see me as the last appointment of the day. She sneaked in the door just as the office was closing, and we sat down and talked about her weight-loss goals. Mary was a well-known public figure whose personal "figure" had grown with weight gain in middle age. In addition to some early health problems of sleep disturbance, rising blood pressure and rising cholesterol, she increasingly felt self-conscious in performing her public duties and making appearances. Mary was also extremely concerned about protecting her privacy. She didn't want to disclose publicly or even privately that she was considering a weight-loss operation.

As we have with some other public figures who sought privacy protections, our office scheduled all of Mary's appointments after hours and scheduled her operation under a pseudonym. Mary underwent a successful outpatient LAP-BAND® procedure at our surgical center and stayed there a grand total of 3-½ hours. She has dropped more than 60 pounds, resolved the cholesterol, blood pressure and sleeping difficulties, and approaches her public responsibilities with greater enthusiasm and nimbleness. Thus far she has not had to disclose her personal decision with anyone publicly. She has begun to do so privately, but on her own timetable.

Make after-hours arrangements. Some practices will accommodate requests for high levels of privacy and discretion by making after-hours appointments. I have done this on a few rare occasions for very well-known politicians and personalities who wanted their decisions kept from the public. There is no guarantee your surgeon will accommodate your desires, but if you think there's a chance you'll be recognized, and the media will be interested in publicizing your personal decisions, it is certainly reasonable to ask for this type of accommodation.

I have seen patients after 5:30 or 6:00 in the evening when nearly all my staff has gone home and there are no patients in the waiting room. While it's not an absolutely foolproof system, it does cut down on the number of people apt to see you coming or going from the weight-loss surgery clinic.

Use a pseudonym. Some practices, hospitals and surgery centers allow you to register under a pseudonym to avoid prying eyes becoming aware of your health or your status as a patient of a practice or facility.

In one case, a prominent physician in my community wanted to keep his weight-loss operation private. We allowed him to use a pseudonym because he was so well-known to all the doctors and nurses, hospital and health care employees in the community that the simple appearance of his name as a patient would have spurred inevitable conversations. A pseudonym served him well, and he shared his decision and the details of his weight-loss journey with only those close to him. (I have noticed that over time he has become a bit more open about it and even shares his decision with patients who are overweight in an attempt to help them understand weight-loss procedures as options for themselves. But it has been totally his choice to disclose this.)

It is your right to decide how much or how little to share with other people. Let your surgeon and the surgery center staff know your preferences and make certain you are satisfied with their ability to honor your wishes. Understand it is nearly impossible to entirely protect privacy in this day and age, but that your surgeon and surgical practice will take every precaution.

Weight-Loss Surgery and Mexico

In recent years a number of people seeking weight-loss procedures have chosen to go outside the country for them. Numerous sites in Mexico and elsewhere now advertise bariatric surgery (usually LAGB) online in an attempt to attract patients to their sunny shores for operations. The primary appeal is lower costs – or at least the possibility of lower costs. But traveling to Mexico for weight-loss surgery doesn't usually make sense.

While the Web sites set up to attract patients to foreign clinics tend to play up lower costs, think for a moment about the importance of the procedure you're considering undergoing. Think about how important the decision and the operation itself are to your life and your well-being.

Keep in mind that most experienced U.S. bariatric surgeons and program directors are very uncomfortable taking on the routine long-term management and band fills of patients who have chosen to go to Mexico for LAGB surgery. The chances of problems are too high, and the liability exposure too great, to justify taking on all the problematic cases done in Mexico. If you have your procedure performed in Mexico and develop complications after your return to the U.S., you may find it very difficult to find a physician willing to treat you in this country.

Is "saving" a few thousand dollars worth the risk? You are considering an operation for long-term results. Will a low-cost version of a procedure give you those results? And consider carefully your health and safety. In the United States, part of the cost of medical care is the cost of oversight placed on surgeons, hospitals and outpatient surgery centers. These people and places are carefully monitored for safety, hygiene and expertise.

There are excellent surgeons and centers outside the United States; there is no question about that. And if you carefully research all the details and know the surgeons and facilities, then it is certainly possible to have a successful LAGB procedure. However, by the same token, I have personally intervened in a number of cases where patients have undergone failed or inappropriately performed weight-loss surgical procedures outside the country. The most recent case was a young woman who lived in Nevada and traveled to Mexico because she could save $4,000. The LAP-BAND® was placed improperly, and she developed a very serious gastric obstruction requiring an emergency operation to correct. And the kicker? Her American insurance company not only wouldn't pay for her Mexican adventure, but they would not pay for any of the hospitalization or surgery required to fix that problem. Now she is paying off bills totaling more than $50,000. Hardly a savings.

> Arriving at one point is the starting point to another.
>
> – JOHN DEWEY

Another case presented at a conference involved a patient who paid money to have a LAP-BAND® procedure in Mexico only to return to the United States with nothing but a few incisions and no actual band placed. What recourse do you have if something like this occurs outside the U.S.?

Think carefully before you decide to leave the country to have LAGB or any other surgical procedure. Ask yourself:

» How much money will I really save?

» Will my insurance company cover me if I have any complications after the procedure?

» Can I find a qualified doctor and bariatric surgeon to take care of me after I return from my out-of-country surgical procedure?

» What is my plan should a complication arise? Will I go back to Mexico, or will I seek a local facility and throw myself on the mercy of the staff?

» Do I have any personal or professional references to recommend the weight-loss surgeon that I am considering seeing outside the United States?

Food for Thought

» Along with the freedom of choice – to choose your surgical weight-loss procedure, your surgeon and your outpatient surgery center – comes the responsibility for your own health, safety and welfare: Do your research thoroughly on each and understand the pros and cons of each choice you make.

» Your top consideration when choosing an outpatient surgery center for your surgical weight-loss procedure is to find a safe, comfortable and professional environment.

» If you prefer the security of a full hospital, keep in mind that every outpatient surgical center has a contingency plan if complications with your procedure arise, and many are physically attached to major hospitals.

» While surgeons recognize that adolescents are still developing psychologically as well as physically, the devastating effects of obesity need to be considered with regard to minimally invasive surgical weight-loss procedures.

» Minimally invasive weight-loss surgical procedures can help older patients lose weight, improve health, increase activities and elevate quality of life. In addition, older patients seem to tolerate the discomfort and inconvenience of the procedures and the accompanying anesthesia better than younger patients.

» Patients over 65 will have a harder time finding a surgeon to perform the procedure for them: Most surgeons and surgical centers will not work with Medicare, and patients over 65 are automatically covered by Medicare.

» More insurance carriers cover weight-loss surgical procedures than ever before, but some still refuse coverage, and some place huge hurdles between the patient and the procedure.

» If you choose to pursue your weight-loss surgical procedure by paying out-of-pocket, you need to be aware additional charges may occur if there are complications with your procedure.

» Many surgical centers offer agreements that allow patients to pay a premium in addition to fees for the procedure in order to cover the costs if complications do arise.

» Whether you choose to tell anyone about the procedure you've chosen to undertake or not is your business. Your surgeon and surgical center will do work to protect your privacy if you choose to keep it secret.

» If you choose not to keep your procedure secret, you may be able to help others with their choices and can also interact more with others who have chosen to have the same procedure or have already done so. There are numerous studies describing the long-term benefits of successful weight loss and most of them point to personal group support as being very important.

» Some people are seeking weight-loss surgical procedures out of the country to minimize costs. While there are some excellent clinics outside the U.S., most surgeons in this country will not work on a patient who is having complications from a surgical procedure performed outside of the U.S. If complications arise after your return, you may find yourself unable to find a qualified surgeon to help you. And you're apt to pay far more correcting complications than you saved in the first place.

'Thought is the sculptor who can create the person you want to be.'

– Henry David Thoreau

5

Getting Ready

HAVING WEIGHT-LOSS SURGERY is a lot more than just walking into the surgery center and going under the knife. It represents a commitment to achieving something important, something very valuable for the long term: Improved health.

Take advantage of the time before your surgery to plan your steps for optimum success. A weight-loss surgical procedure can be a powerful tool in your effort to lose weight and keep it off. But the surgery does not work all by itself – it takes hard work and commitment to success to achieve the kind of amazing weight loss possible when you set your mind to it and prepare.

Preoperative Phase

Once you've made the decision to proceed with a weight-loss operation and made your choice whether to keep your decision a secret or share it as you see fit, you're entering the preoperative phase of weight loss.

At this point you'll be working with a weight-loss program through the surgeon's practice. If you have insurance, the program you're working with will be in the process of obtaining pre-approval on the procedure. Meanwhile, you'll be working on additional steps required by the program. Most likely these steps are going to involve consultations with a psychologist, a nutritionist or dietician, and often they will involve attending some support groups.

For some people this all feels intrusive. They've made the decision to proceed, and now that's exactly what they want to do – proceed. Others use this time for exactly what it is meant for – education and growth. With a couple months to go before the operation, this is a time for learning everything possible, a time for maximum education about the whole process, the entire weight-loss journey.

Books

To begin with, I think it's a terrific idea to buy a book or two on the subject. That way you'll understand things that might not have made sense to you when they were explained in the sometimes intimidating clinical setting, and you can look up answers to sudden questions that occur to you at 4 a.m. when your surgeon is at home, asleep, not available to answer them.

There are several good texts out there on bariatric surgery, including *Weight Loss Surgery for Dummies* by Kurian, Thompson and Davidson and *Bariatric Support: Crossing Over to a New You*, by Williamson. And soon there will be a new text, a Comprehensive Sasse Guide to Surgical Weight Loss.

Audio CDs and Audio MP3 Programs

Feed your brain with some positive messages and valuable tips about weight-loss success, health and fitness. It is said that we are exposed to more than 20,000 messages about food, sweets and carbohydrates during the course of the year. Think of the billboards, TV commercials and radio ads your senses take in every day. How many of those are telling your brain you should eat more goodies and load up on calories? That's right – a lot of them.

You can change the messages your brain receives by going out and finding some high-quality audio programs that promote good scientific principles and techniques for eating healthier and becoming fitter. Listen in your car, while you exercise or just play them at home. I have prepared several audio programs that cover technical aspects of weight-loss surgery and the surgeon's role in detail, discuss recovery time and how to maximize recovery and minimize downtime. And they explore in more detail what you can do to maximize your weight-loss success during the first six months and beyond. Visit *www.AudioDiets.com* to check out some of these audio programs that could really help you maximize your weight-loss success and reinforce sound principles of weight-loss and health.

Support Groups

It's an excellent idea to start attending support group meetings at your bariatric surgical center on a regular basis. At Western Bariatric, we offer weekly groups, with many different groups in different parts of town, so in our area it's easy to find one that fits a patient's schedule and geographic location. Your surgeon's office will know what support groups are available in your area.

Support groups serve a number of purposes. In addition to fulfilling the important goal of learning about the weight-loss operation you're going to undergo, a group offers a place where you can meet people who are also about to embark on the same journey you're going to follow, and those people who have already started. You'll meet patients and their loved ones who are at the same point in the process that you are, as well as those in different places. And you can make friends with people who have had common problems and now have common goals.

Support groups present opportunities to ask questions about the experiences of people who have already had their operations.

You can ask questions you were too embarrassed to ask your surgeon or nursing staff or that you just keep forgetting to ask. You can ask questions your surgeon might not be able to answer because the surgeon hasn't experienced the operation from the inside out – unlike the person standing in front of you at a support group.

You may also meet people at support groups whose recoveries didn't go so smoothly. While nine times out of 10 weight-loss surgery goes as planned with no complications or problems, if you meet someone whose operation was difficult you have a chance to ask some questions. What were the complications? How did they happen? Was the surgeon caring, conscientious and committed to making sure there was a successful outcome? This is valuable information from people whose journeys may have diverged from the path yours will most likely take in the hands of an experienced surgeon.

Preoperative Classes

Preoperative classes will vary from program to program. But on the whole, most weight-loss programs will include a series of classes aimed at providing additional tools for long-term weight-loss success.

Patient Story: Katie S.

Procedure: **LRYGB**
Weight lost: **130 pounds**

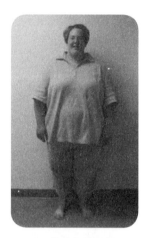

Katie before

I was 34 years old and felt like I was going on 60 years old! I was short of breath, I had high blood pressure, depression, sleep apnea, pre-diabetes, sore/achy muscles and bones, and that was just the physical! Emotionally, I was self-conscious, embarrassed by the way I looked and how I dressed. I was frustrated by the fact that I couldn't run and play and do things with my children. I was living a vicious circle. I wanted to exercise but was too fat and unhealthy. I was afraid of dying of a heart attack, and it literally hurt. If I didn't exercise, I would never be healthy.

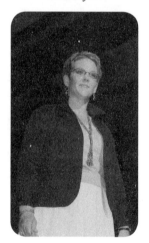

Katie after

I really wanted to lose weight without surgery, but I had failed so many times on diets, and I felt like my life was passing me by, and I wasn't living, I was dying. It took me five years to finally have the courage to have the surgery. Then I was denied by my insurance. My surgeon was wonderful and challenged the insurance and got the surgery covered.

I was very nervous about having to give up food. Food was a joy to me. I loved eating, loved the taste, smell, everything. I hated the sensation of being hungry. I was hoping that the surgery would help me feel full sooner and relieve the pain of hunger.

The surgery was fine. My pain medication didn't work in the hospital, but once I was on liquid pain medicine, I did great! I was very compliant. I did everything that I was asked to do. I am now two and a half years post surgery and my "dumping syndrome" has diminished. I can eat everything except ice cream and milk shakes. I still "dump" when I eat more than about 20 grams of sugar. I can eat more, but I have to be very careful. I now have to worry about gaining the weight back. I have never touched soda pop, coffee, tea or alcohol since surgery. I use my surgery as a tool. I still can't eat as much as I could before surgery.

I did not take the decision to have this surgery lightly, and I would not recommend it to someone that could not be disciplined enough to handle it. I plan on continuing my weight loss. I did have a baby seven months ago and gained a little, but have every intention to continue losing.

This surgery changed my life and was the best decision I have ever made.

One thing you have to remember: Weight-loss procedures don't work in a vacuum. The operation is not a miracle cure that works solely by itself. Weight-loss procedures work *with you.*

That's one of the first things I tell patients. No surgery works by itself. No surgery is foolproof. Every surgery can be undermined. There is no operation that can be done that will guarantee success in the long term. The only thing that is absolutely definitive in predicting success is *your total and complete commitment to success.*

If you can commit to making your weight-loss operation a success, if you've done your homework, found the right surgeon, and you are willing to do the work before and after the operation, you've got a fantastic chance of success.

But a person *can* fail. Any patient can have a successful operation and a lousy weight-loss program due to eating the wrong foods, avoiding exercise, failing to work on better habits and not making the right food choices. And that would be sad after there's been so much time and energy and money devoted to the weight-loss procedure, and so much hope derailed. One way to avoid failing after going to all the time and effort of having a weight-loss procedure is to take advantage of the classes, support groups, audio programs and books available with expert advice, guidance and motivation along the way – your goals are too important not to utilize everything in your favor!

For most people considering a weight-loss operation, the effort to lose weight in the past has been an uphill battle. Many people have had transient successes followed by long periods of failure and gradual weight gain over the years. But after their operations those same people now find that with their continuing efforts the battle is easily won. The pounds come off as never before, and better still, *they stay off.*

So, while surgery is not a silver bullet that magically results in weight loss, it is a highly effective weapon in the battle against those unwanted pounds. I often tell my patients that the operation will be a very potent weapon in the battle to lose weight – but it won't fight the battle *all by itself.* If you want the procedure to change your life, you have to participate; you have to make healthy food choices, exercise and stay focused on the goals of becoming healthier, fitter and happier.

What to Expect in Your Preoperative Months

In our program, the first several preoperative classes emphasize the importance of personal responsibility in succeeding in the weight-loss journey. The classes that follow offer dietary counseling, a good deal of education about nutrition and the kind of calorie count we're looking for, explanations of what an energy deficit is and discussion of what sort of energy content is present with protein and with carbohydrates and with fat and alcohol.

> The first problem for all of us, men and women, is not to learn, but to unlearn.
>
> – GLORIA STEINEM

The next step of our preoperative program covers fitness and exercise and the important parts both play in weight-loss success. Fitness trainers contribute to the classes and prepare instructional materials and demonstrations. Participants get log books, pedometers, educational handouts and other supplies to help them on their road to healthier lives. A chef comes in to talk about cooking and provides valuable insight and cooking and shopping demonstrations (shopping demonstrations might seem unnecessary, but how many times have you gone home with an unintended bag of chips or gallon of ice cream?)

All of these elements form the backbone of the comprehensive long-term weight-loss strategy. These classes take place during that interim period between the time you've made the decision to avail yourself of a life-changing weight-loss procedure and the time you actually have your operation.

Education is one of the keys to successful long-term weight loss, and it's available to you in quantity during this time. I highly recommend you take advantage of it.

Preoperative Liquid Diet

Approximately four weeks before your operation the staff at many weight-loss programs, including ours at Western Bariatric Institute, will ask you to change to a liquid protein diet. You'll be getting your daily calories from liquid meal-replacement protein shakes, which do facilitate weight loss. (*See Appendix B*)

You may be wondering why you need to do this if you're having a weight-loss operation. There are several reasons, including the jump-start it gives you on weight loss after your procedure and the fact that losing weight before your operation makes for a safer procedure.

One of the critical reasons is to shrink the liver. In the last few years, data has proven that the liver shrinks disproportionately to anything else in the abdomen when one follows a protein-based liquid meal-replacement system for two weeks. Studies using MRI scanners and laparoscopy evaluations demonstrated the extent to which the liver shrank.[31]

Fine, you think, I want to lose weight, not have smaller organs. Actually, in this instance you do want smaller organs. During surgery, we sometimes have difficulty with very large fatty-infiltrated livers. The liver, and specifically the left lobe of the liver, has to be moved out of the way to give us access to the upper part of the stomach. If the liver is very large it has a tendency to crack, which can cause bleeding and complications. Sometimes this leads to changing a laparoscopic surgery to open surgery with all the attendant risks and complications: infections, hernias and prolonged hospital stays, to name a few.

So, something as simple as going on a four-week preoperative liquid meal-replacement diet can make a dramatic difference in the whole weight-loss operation experience. We have worked to make this liquid diet program more fun and more palatable by asking world-renowned chef Dave Fouts to prepare a recipe book of protein shakes. The recipes in Chef Dave's book, *Shakin' It Up*, offer plenty of tasty options for the liquid diet. (You can order this book and others at *www.iMetabolic.com*. *See Appendix B for sample recipes and details on how to order Chef Dave's books.*)

We started instituting a practice of the two-week liquid meal-replacement phase in 2006 and found the results were striking. Patients whose cases might once have caused us to expect to contend with large livers or cracked livers and bleeding complications or cases in which we might even have had to abort surgery because of a liver that was just too large were now no problem.

Last year we increased the program to four weeks, with fantastic results (and some centers insist on as long as six, eight or even 12 weeks). Since this change we very rarely find complications due to overly large livers, because everyone goes on the preoperative liquid meal-replacement program, and pretty much everybody has nicely shrunken livers. Not every patient complies with the program, and not every liver shrinks the way we'd like it to, but for the most part, by the time the operation takes place, most people's livers have shrunken. While it's nice for surgeons not to have to contend with oversized livers, it's nice for patients, too – it makes for a smoother operation with fewer chances of complications and easier recoveries because we didn't have to drag a large liver out of the way.

Mark

I saw Mark in follow-up recently after his surgery. Mark had done very well initially after an outpatient LAGB procedure, but he struggled in his ongoing battle to lose more weight. Starting at 295 pounds, Mark lost 24 pounds during the preoperative weight-loss phase. So, he had a good initial jumping off point. His surgery went very smoothly, and he initially lost an additional 10 pounds in the first month. Over the course of the next eight months, Mark lost an additional 25 pounds, so that he then weighed 235 pounds, 59 pounds down from his original weight.

Mark's goal, however, had been to reach a weight of 190 pounds, where he felt the most comfortable. He had the LAP-BAND® adjusted several times and complained that the band always seemed to be either too tight or too loose. After several of these trials of adding and subtracting minute amounts of saline from the band, I counseled Mark that the problem did not reside with the band. The LAP-BAND®, I told him, is merely a tool and an imperfect one at that. It does provide him some degree of improved satiety and better appetite control. It also "puts on the brakes" for Mark when he might otherwise overeat. But it is certainly not a foolproof or magically effective device that results in effortless, unlimited weight loss.

More recently Mark has had some success transitioning to a focus on more sustained and regular exercise, and on developing and maintaining long-term successful habits such as eating a low-calorie, low glycemic-index breakfast every morning consisting of a shake or bar that is based on protein and vitamins. Eating breakfast allows Mark's body to kick-start his metabolism and results in the burning of more consumed calories during the day. Mark has continued to lose weight slowly and is taking more responsibility for his long-term weight loss.

But smaller livers is not the only reason surgical practices have instituted weeks-long preoperative liquid meal-replacement programs. Such programs are an excellent way to begin weight loss. Induction or initiation diets kick off nonsurgical medically supervised rapid weight-loss programs beginning with liquid protein replacement shakes and lead to very rapid weight loss. We're doing a miniature version of those programs.

What happens with these rapid weight-loss liquid-diet programs is that people tend to lose two to four pounds a week. In some cases, patients who are starting out with a great deal of weight to lose may lose as much as six to eight pounds a week on a very low calorie liquid meal-replacement diet. With weight loss like this, in a very short amount of time you can lose 15 or 18 pounds with the initial weight loss achieved with very small intervention and very profound results. This helps start off the weight loss both physically and mentally – there's nothing like losing 15 pounds in a very short time to make weight loss seem like a real-world possibility. And if you're losing the weight as a precursor to a surgical weight-loss procedure, those are pounds you're likely never going to see again. It feels good.

In addition to all the other benefits, losing even 10 or 15 pounds before an operation makes going under anesthesia safer. It makes postoperative recovery easier because you have less weight to carry around, less body mass restricting movements of the chest, so breathing is easier, and oxygenation of the blood is easier. Really, the weight loss favorably effects virtually every organ system.

Want even more good news? We have found that people taking medications for blood pressure and diabetes can lose enough weight on the preoperative meal-replacement program that their blood pressure and blood sugar normalize, again making the upcoming operation that much safer.

So, there are a number of reasons the preoperative liquid meal-replacement diet is important, and I urge you to talk to your surgeon about it and to comply rigorously with your surgeon's recommendations.

Most people find the diet isn't that hard to follow. During the first couple days using only liquid shakes people get pretty hungry, and if they're not committed it's easy to fall off the program and eat something not on the recommended menu. But by the third, fourth or fifth day, most people find their bodies and appetites have adjusted. An intrinsic kind of appetite suppression seems to kick in and most people feel perfectly satisfied with the shakes alone. So, stick with it through the first critical days, and you'll find it becomes much easier, and you'll reap the benefits with rapid weight loss and a healthier body for your weight-loss operation.

Exercise

If you thought you were just going to spend the time between deciding on a weight-loss procedure and actually having it undergoing a few medical tests and waiting for insurance forms, think again. Not only are you going to be dieting and learning and going to support groups, but this is a great time to start exercising. You're preparing for your new life, and if you really want to succeed in that life you're going to have to make exercise a part of it. Starting *before* your weight-loss procedure just gives you a head start.

As with losing weight and dieting and shrinking your liver and reducing some of your risks from health problems, exercise can reduce your risk levels for the operation.

First off, surgical procedures are stressful. They're hard on the body, like any physical endeavor, and just because the operation is done to you rather than you doing it doesn't make it less stressful. If you can improve your physical condition – get stronger, improve your cardiovascular system – you improve your chances of coming through without complications.

Before a weight-loss operation you want to start an exercise program that will help you improve your conditioning, your cardiovascular status, your stamina, your strength and your endurance, all of which will help you move through your operation much more easily. Studies have shown that some of the specific pulmonary mechanics, the numerical measures of the effectiveness of your lungs, are significantly improved by preoperative exercise programs – that's exactly what you're looking for. [89, 90]

If that's not enough, exercise can help you feel better emotionally about your upcoming operation and it can improve your sleep. Not to mention exercise can also help you attain weight loss before your operation by increasing the calories you burn, thus lowering your risks further.

> The thing always happens that you really believe in; and the belief in a thing makes it happen.
>
> – FRANK LLOYD WRIGHT

What kind of exercise should you do? That depends on you and what you like, but in general you should pick something you're comfortable with, something you enjoy doing and something you can sustain long-term. In many cases people choose to start with taking brisk walks. For people who have trouble with walking because of joint or back pain, exercise bikes, elliptical trainers and exercising in pools doing water aerobics (or one of many other exercises available today) may be better choices. Your exercise program might involve something as simple as buying five- or 10-pound hand weights and vigorously exercising your arms while you're at rest even if you can't do much in the way of walking or standing.

But whatever you pick, it's helpful to start now and to keep at it every day.

Don't know how to start? Your surgery center staff should have some ideas. At Western Bariatric Institute we provide ideas about exercise for every patient who walks through our door, whether or not the person decides on a weight-loss operation or chooses to work with a nonsurgical alternative.

For starters, all patients get pedometers so they can monitor how many steps they're taking in an average day. With the exception of those patients who have joint problems or problems walking, most people can and should add more steps to their daily routines.

Walking not only burns calories, it improves physical conditioning and helps prepare the body for the operation. Start with a goal of taking 8,000 steps every day. When that becomes easy, increase the goal to 10,000 and then 12,000. Our patients find with time and commitment and motivation they will hit their goals and head into their operations in much better shape than when they started with the extra steps.

Attitude

I'd also like to suggest positive imaging. I know that might sound a little too much like new-age thinking for some readers, the idea that you can think positively and prepare psychologically for physical outcomes, but there is a good body of data supporting the idea that thinking positively and indulging in some creative positive mental imagery may improve the outcomes of an operation. So, as you learn more and read more and talk to more people as you get closer to the date of your weight-loss procedure, take some time to sit down and think through the experience and imagine all of it going smoothly and very positively.

Imagine yourself coming in for the operation, meeting the people who are going to be taking care of you, having very positive experiences with them. Visualize the operation going smoothly and see yourself coming out of anesthesia without significant pain and without nausea or side effects, and see yourself recovering with very little pain or discomfort. Visualize yourself embarking on the hard work to come while feeling energized and confident. As you continue to work with these positive images I think you'll find that you're setting the stage for the kind of positive experience with weight loss that you want.

How Much Time Off Will I Need?

You're going to want to ask your surgeon that, of course. But while different surgeons hold differing opinions on time off, there are some general guidelines.

First, you're probably planning to undergo a laparoscopic weight-loss procedure. With rare exceptions there is really no good reason for having an open surgical procedure unless you've had a great number of previous abdominal operations or had a previous gastric bypass procedure or there is some other very unusual set of circumstances. (Multiple previous abdominal operations means a high chance of extensive intra-abdominal adhesions or scar tissue. This scar tissue can make laparoscopic surgery impossible.) But for 98 percent of us, weight-loss procedures mean laparoscopic or minimally invasive procedures with keyhole incisions.

Assuming you're having a minimally invasive operation, one to two weeks off is a good ballpark. This is too much for some people and not enough for others, but it gives you an average. If your job requires heavy lifting or a lot of activity, you might want to take three or four weeks off. And it doesn't hurt to have a cushion so if complications occur you can take longer for recovery. But the amount of time you can take depends on your situation and your job and also whether or not you've disclosed the nature of your absence or kept your weight-loss operation plans to yourself.

Over the years I've seen many patients go back to their jobs, especially office jobs, within a matter of days. One patient who was an employee at my practice had a laparoscopic RYGB operation on Monday and came back to work on Thursday. I tried to convince her not to, but she actually seemed fine, physically, and it was important to her psychologically.

One of my colleagues at the hospital had an LAGB procedure one day and returned to his full duties the next day. So, it depends a lot on your motivation, your comfort level and your attitude.

Some people find they tire quickly and are more fatigued at the end of the day even after the recovery period. It can take a good six to eight weeks to get back to normal energy levels, but this is true of all kinds of operations and minor procedures. Medical science doesn't know exactly why this is, but it may have something to do with the stress of surgical procedures, anesthesia and recovery. It's simply a good thing to know and plan around so that you're not following up your operation with 12- and 14-hour days. Try to take off for two weeks, for certain, with the option of working a lighter schedule or being able to get extra rest during the weeks that follow.

It's also important to make sure you have a safety net if you have children or parents to care for. During the weeks leading up to your operation try to line up other people who can pitch in and take over these responsibilities. If you're the one who usually does the shopping and cleaning, you may want to even hire somebody to come in and help. You really need to give yourself time to focus on just you and your recovery.

The Countdown

One Month Prior to Your Procedure

Along with the physical changes you're making before your operation and everything you're learning, this is a good time to sit down and talk with your loved ones about the journey you are embarking upon. You may have decided not to tell many people that you're going to undergo a weight-loss operation, but you probably need to have a core group of people close to you who will be supportive and there to help you along your journey. Talk to these people about what you're doing and, if you're comfortable doing so, share your hopes and dreams and goals for the operation with your friends and loved ones.

This is a good time to help those people who are close to you understand how important a step this is for you. Explain that this is something you have decided to undertake in order to live a healthier, better quality and longer life and that you're looking forward to spending time with them, maybe enjoying outdoor activities with family and friends or working on alleviating health problems you've begun to experience. Or tell them that you are working to make sure you don't succumb to the type of health problems that nagged your relatives or stopped your parents from living the lives they wanted to live.

Define Your Goals

You may have other goals that family and friends don't suspect. Maybe there's a hidden athlete inside you. Maybe you want to go rafting with the family next summer or climb a mountain. Maybe you have goals about your physical appearance. If you're not comfortable sharing your goals with others, review them when you have some time alone. Make a list of the things you want to do after your operation. Remind yourself of all the reasons you've sought a weight-loss procedure – for your health, for your longevity, for a chance to spend more time doing more of the activities you enjoy with your loved ones.

Write down your goals. Put them on your mirror or other places where you'll see them often and remember that what you're doing is embarking on a very important journey. It's very important for your long-term health and your long-term quality of life. And your long-term life.

The last month before your operation is a good time to attend preoperative classes and support groups. It's also time to review the things that need to be done before your operation. Double-check with your program that insurance authorization is under-way. Make sure you have childcare or eldercare set up for the first week or two after your surgery when you're going to need a little extra time and assistance yourself.

Also, if you haven't done so, this is the time for two important steps that are required by all the national Centers of Excellence from the American Society of Bariatric Surgery and increasingly by insurance companies: the meetings with the dietician or nutri-tionist, and a meeting with a psychologist (at least one meeting is required; others are optional.)

Take advantage of these opportunities. I know some patients view them as simply more boxes to be checked off while getting ready for the operation and find them a bit of an annoyance, but many people find these visits very, very valuable.

Psychological Evaluation

At Western Bariatric Institute we work with a panel of psychol-ogists who have become very experienced at offering preopera-tive assessments and counseling for people undergoing weight-loss procedures. They are experts in behavior modification and in all aspects of the psychology of the weight-loss journey.

Sitting down with a psychologist before your weight-loss operation can be very valuable. The psychologist is there to offer some insight to you about what will work for you to succeed and what things you might think about to help you on your journey. The psychologist is also there, in part, to assess your suitability and candidacy for a weight-loss procedure. Insurance companies are in the habit of requiring a psychologist's approval before authorizing surgery, so this visit is usually one on the checklist of things to do before surgery is officially scheduled. This isn't a cause for concern – very few candidates are turned away on the basis of psychological evaluations, though some candidates are found to have deeper emotional issues that require some counseling or treatment prior to and after surgery. Identifying these concerns ahead of time will only improve the surgical outcome.

This doesn't mean you have gone into therapy or that anyone will know that you have seen a psychologist. But, if you do have ongoing concerns as you make the transitions in your life that a weight-loss procedure brings about, many of these professionals are willing to work with weight-loss patients on an ongoing basis.

Most of the changes from weight-loss procedures are positive, but some can be stressful. Changes in body image and how other people react to you and treat you can be a new stress in your life. Or weight loss may result in new attention from others, which can be stressful if it's unexpected. A psychologist can help you through your transitions or, if you're only working with the psychologist before the operation, help you prepare. So, the psychological evaluation is a valuable opportunity to learn more and interact with an experienced professional in the field of surgical weight loss.

Evaluation

The same is true for the dietary or the nutritional consultation. At Western Bariatric Institute, typically about 90 percent of patients will see one of four dietitians who perform the bulk of the nutritional evaluations prior to operations. Our dietitians are invested in seeing patients succeed. They're advocates of the surgical weight-loss process and have seen a great number of people come through and dramatically change their lives for the better.

But it's natural to feel a bit apprehensive before visiting with a dietitian. By the time people are contemplating weight-loss procedures, they've already dealt with a good many people in their lives telling them what's what in weight loss, what to do, eat and think. Going to a dietitian when you're already overweight might feel threatening. It's natural to anticipate being told "no, wrong, bad." But it's not going to happen. Our dietitians are interested in your long-term health and well-being, and they're also interested in making sure you have realistic goals and a good understanding of the responsibility that you need to take for long-term success. Dietitians can offer some tremendous insights and ongoing counseling in terms of what foods are good choices for the long term.

PreOP Liquid Diet

The dieticians often play a role in the all-important preoperative liquid meal-replacement diet that you should begin at this point. Your program staff will most likely have already given you details about it, and their version of this preop diet may be somewhat different from what I have outlined in Appendix B. The key is to markedly reduce calories, emphasize protein drinks, plenty of water, exercise and fiber.

Our dietitians meet with patients and perform evaluations and offer insights and suggestions, and they also teach some of the preoperative classes, which give you more chances to interact and ask questions about nutrition and good food choices – tools necessary for long-term success.

We use the protein-based liquid meal-replacement program because we've found people succeed when we take all other choices away. You don't have to worry about what you're going to eat or drink during these last four weeks before your weight-loss surgery because it's all based on liquid shakes and liquid meal replacements. There isn't anything else.

I'll admit my outstanding dietitian, Vicki Bovee, and I fight about whether or not to let people have a bit of steamed broccoli every now and then, and I know she tells them to go ahead and do that if they're just dying for something to eat. It adds a little crunchiness and some additional nutrients without adding too many calories. But typically, I tell people to just stick with the liquid shakes and to not add even the vegetables. Vegetables may not hurt much, but they open the door to temptation.

Online Education

In addition to in-person preoperative classes, there are online classes available from most programs. WBI subscribes to a professionally produced program that is password-protected and has educational modules for the LRYGB, the LAGB and soon, the LSG procedures. These are classes you can view in your own time and at your own pace, so that you may be certain you understand each part before going on.

Liquid Meal Replacements

The fact that you've been following a liquid meal-replacement diet during your preop month doesn't mean you're going to stay on it forever. The liquid meal replacements work very well. They help you focus on your intake of protein, vitamins and fluid, and help you avoid everything else that could be detrimental to losing weight. They can play a helpful role in long-term weight loss, and can easily be prepared for breakfast or lunch, taking the place of a meal, especially one that might be high in carbohydrates. They're also a great snack, taking away hunger and replacing possible extra carbs with proteins and helping you keep your weight down.

But they're not a complete or permanent solution, and you're not expected to continue the liquid meal replacement diet forever. The months before surgery are the time to reshape how you think about food and to learn how to make healthier food choices. This is one place the nutritionist involved with your weight-loss program can definitely help out. Over the long term, you can use the shakes or bars for snacks or breakfast or when you need to refocus your weight loss and avoid a relapse of weight gain.

You'll need to set aside time for all your necessary appointments, and it might seem like there's a lot going on prior to your weight-loss operation – because there is. Take advantage of all the resources available. The more you learn, the better you'll succeed.

Two Weeks Prior to Your Procedure

Two weeks before your operation it doesn't seem like there's much left to do. By now you've had time to talk with your loved ones and support people, hopefully you've attended some preoperative classes, and your insurance authorization is underway. The date of your operation should already be set by now and circled on the calendar. What's left to do?

For one thing, if you haven't already started the preoperative protein-based liquid meal-replacement program, start immediately. If the center you've chosen doesn't offer this kind of program, take a look around at some other centers and see if you can make sense of the programs they're offering.

You can also visit *www.iMetabolic.com* and order protein meal-replacement products that will allow you to put together your own two-week program. That way you've still got time to achieve the results that patients do at the centers that employ this kind of program.

If your program does prescribe a meal replacement program, then stick to it religiously. You want to begin making some changes in your diet and in your way of thinking about food and drink that you will want to sustain for the long term, and these can start with the liquid meal-replacement program.

During this time you're also going to pay strict attention to what you drink. Some programs rule out all carbonated beverages, but I don't think a little carbonation prior to your operation is going to hurt. Just make sure whatever you choose is a zero-calorie drink.

There are a wide variety of zero-calorie beverages on the market today, from Diet Snapple to Diet 7UP. I do advise against drinking caffeinated beverages, simply because of the diuretic effect, which can cause some dehydration. After an operation, many people feel you shouldn't drink carbonated beverages anymore, but I have several personal friends who have had LRYGB and LAGB procedures, and they are able to drink carbonated beverages without too much trouble.

Herbal Remedies

This is also the time to discontinue herbal medications, supplements or remedies you may be taking. Many people don't regard herbal products as medicines and forget to tell their doctors about them. In recent years research has uncovered dangerous side effects of common herbal products in people who are undergoing surgical procedures.[91-92]

It is very important to tell your doctor about herbal medicines you are taking. Many people are unaware that quite a few herbal or so-called "natural" remedies have serious side effects including bleeding. (The American Society of Anesthesiology recommends every patient stop all herbal remedies two to three weeks prior to an operation because of side effects.)

Garlic, ginseng and ginkgo biloba have all been shown to increase bleeding. Kava can increase the sedative effect of anesthetics. Ma huang (ephedra) increases blood pressure and heart rate. Saint-John's-wort alters an important enzyme of the liver that metabolizes many drugs. So, reduce the risks for your operation. Tell the doctor about any of these herbal products and discontinue them for the next two weeks.

At two weeks out from your operation you should be up to 8,000 or even 10,000 steps a day on your pedometer, and be attending preoperative classes. You've probably picked up a couple books on bariatric surgery and want to finish them before the date of your operation. You've talked to loved ones and tried some positive visualization. What else?

For one thing, you need to make sure you've set aside enough time for your recovery. Make certain all arrangements are in place for your time off work. You don't need last-minute panics cropping up or people asking if they can e-mail you or call you, especially if you haven't revealed that you're going to be gone for a weight-loss operation rather than a trip. Childcare arrangements should be double- and triple-checked, and if you're taking care of a parent or older loved one, make sure you've got arrangements for someone to take over that caretaking responsibility as well. You don't want to spend the time just before your operation stressed out, making arrangements, and if you have to cancel or postpone your operation, your surgeon may not be able to accommodate you in your preferred time frame. You've worked hard to get here – now you need to make sure that hard work all pays off.

One Week Prior to Your Procedure

Most practices recommend you stop any medications that cause blood thinning prior to an operation. If you're taking prescribed blood thinners like Coumadin, it's important to discuss that with your surgeon long before your operation (*see Chapter 3*). Typically your surgeon will recommend you go off Coumadin for a period of five to seven days before your operation. In some cases, the surgeon may make additional arrangements for you to be on another kind of blood thinner, though most of the time the decision is to simply stop the blood thinner prior to surgery.

For milder prescribed blood thinners, including aspirin, ibuprofen or naproxen, this is something to cover with your surgeon individually. In my practice, we generally have a standard recommendation to stop these medications five to seven days prior to an operation, but there are times when people need to stay on them. In such cases, it's really up to each individual surgeon to make the call. In my practice, if people have a strong reason to stay on their aspirin or ibuprofen, I let them stay on because I think the risk of bleeding is quite small. But there may be other surgeons who would recommend stopping them altogether. It's a matter for you to discuss with your surgeon.

Usually your surgeon will ask that you visit the hospital or surgery center around a week before your operation to register and go over paperwork, and to have some preoperative tests. (More tests? Yes, I'm afraid so.) These last-minute tests usually include an EKG, a chest X-ray and some blood work. Even if you've had all these done before, they're usually required again close to the operation date so that the results are up-to-date and reflect your health status as you undergo anesthesia and the operation.

Two Days Prior to Your Procedure

Okay, this might sound crazy, but the most important thing to do two days out from your operation date is triple-confirm the date and time and location of the operation.

It sounds silly. But imagine the huge stress it would cause if it turned out you were planning on going to the wrong place at the wrong time on the wrong day – or any of the above. Figuring it out at the last minute might save the surgery, but it will cause you to be stressed and rushed, which is not the experience you want to have.

So, two days before the operation, confirm exactly where you're supposed to be and when, and take the time to double-check with the people who are going to help you the day of your operation.

Support Team

For some people, as many as two or three support people might be necessary, but one intelligent, supportive person is often the right number. This is the person who is going with you to the hospital or outpatient center and who will accompany you through your journey.

I think it's very helpful to have your support person or team with you to hear everything the doctors and nurses tell you before and after your operation. Someone who is not undergoing the procedure is probably going to be a little more relaxed and might ask better questions and retain more of the information. Then that person can help you through those first days after your operation when you're apt to be sore and need the most assistance.

Typically, it's going to be a spouse or best friend who will support you through the weight-loss operation, driving you to the facility, remaining through the procedure, listening to the information from doctors and nurses and seeing you home again. A few days prior to your operation is a good time to discuss with your support person or team exactly what's going to take place and what you should all prepare for.

In the case of LAGB procedures, 80 to 90 percent of procedures can be done in outpatient facilities. So, your support person is going to bring you to the facility early in the morning, most likely, and help you prepare for your operation. Your support person can stay while you have your IV placed, move with you to the preoperative area and meet with the surgeon and wait during the operation. After your operation your support person will meet with the surgeon again, and, after your recovery period, take you back home.

If your support person can spend the night with you after you return home, so much the better, and it wouldn't hurt to have support for the next couple days. Most people don't need someone to wait on them hand and foot, but it's nice to have someone who can do the cooking, bring you things to drink or read or extra pillows and walk with you when you're not walking at your usual brisk pace and need someone with a little extra patience. While most people are physically capable of going it alone after most outpatient surgeries, I don't think there's anything more valuable than having a best friend or partner who can be around for a few days. After the first couple days you'll probably feel more like yourself, but in the beginning it's nice to have the support.

If you're having an LRYGB procedure, the advice is a little different. You should expect an overnight hospital stay, or even two nights (at our center it seems to be split evenly between one- and two-night stays). With rare occurrences, the stay can be longer, three or four nights, or in rare cases of complications, longer than that.

The Day Prior to Your Procedure

Some people want to go out for one last big meal, a celebratory blowout, and, in Nevada, where I practice, the casinos have big, beautiful buffets that can be really tempting. But your blowout could blow it, ruining the two-week or longer meal-replacement diet you've been carefully following and probably making you feel worse than you might expect. I strongly advise against this.

The day before your procedure is a good day to review what you're going to be doing the following day, review where you're going to be and when you need to be there, make sure your support person is up to date with your plans and double-check that your rides are arranged.

The day before your operation is a good day to have quiet at home. It's a good day to reflect on your goals, to look at the progress you've made so far, to visualize a successful outcome to the operation coming up and daydream about the new life your future holds.

Some programs have preoperative medications or preoperative bowel preparation or cleansing, so you might end up taking the entire day off work. Your surgeon will give you specific instructions, as different programs use different procedures. At our center, we recommend a bowel cleanse for all patients undergoing LRYGB surgery or complex revision procedures but not for LAGB, LSG or StomaphyX™. While not critical to the success of the operation, the bowel preparation does empty out the intestinal system and can help reduce postoperative constipation, bloating and even infection. In the early days of gastric bypass, there was a chance of bowel perforation and contamination, and the risk of infection was lowered by cleansing out the bowels ahead of time. Today, experienced laparoscopic surgeons almost never encounter that type of problem, and, as a result, most centers have dropped the requirement of the bowel preparation except for with LRYGB.

The day prior to your operation is a good day for long, brisk walks, for continuing your exercise program and for taking care of any last minute arrangements you need to make. Set aside time for a good night's sleep.

Generally speaking, if you're taking medications for ongoing health conditions, such as heart conditions, high blood pressure or any other significant medical conditions that require ongoing medication, you should continue to take your medicines the day before your operation. In most cases, we actually recommend patients take them the morning of an operation, but only with the smallest sip of water. We want the stomach as empty as possible for the procedure.

Diabetes

People with diabetes – a fairly common medical condition in patients considering weight-loss procedures – are the exception to the medications rule, as the need for medications to control the condition has likely dropped over the previous several weeks. On the day before your operation, if you've been following the preoperative meal-replacement diet, your blood sugars should have fallen (your medication requirements, should you have any, have probably fallen also in the last four weeks). So, if you have diabetes, the day before your operation, when you're having your meal-replacement shake again and nothing else, you may not need much in terms of insulin or oral medication due to the cumulative impact of your meal-replacement plan.

Keep a watch on your blood sugar. Try to target a range of 120 to 150. It's okay if it creeps a little higher, you just don't want it to fall too far below 100, because you don't want it to really bottom out and be in the dangerous 50 to 60 range the night or morning of your operation. Remember, you won't be eating anything the next morning, so let it drift up a little.

If you do take insulin regularly for diabetes, most practices and most endocrinologists recommend you take only half the normal dose the evening before your surgery. You're not going to even have a protein shake or a cup of coffee the morning of your operation. The most you're going to have is a sip of water to wash down any regular important medications.

The Day of Your Procedure

Welcome to the day of your operation. You've worked long and hard to get here. There are only a few more steps.

First thing: Don't eat. The number-one reason operations get canceled at the last minute is that the patient had something to eat or too much to drink. In that case the anesthesiologist is faced with a person who is significantly overweight and also has what is referred to in anesthesia as a "full stomach." Full-stomach anesthesia is only performed in emergencies when there's no choice – and weight-loss surgery is not a trauma situation, nor should it be. A full stomach causes too high a risk of aspiration, where stomach contents can come upward and be breathed into the lungs.

You've worked so hard and taken all the trouble to arrange time off and put together a support team and arranged childcare and everything else you've done in the last two months, it would be a shame to waste it. So put nothing in your stomach the morning of your operation but your prescribed medications with a sip of water.

You'll probably want to bring your CD player or your iPod with you and a book or magazine, because inevitably we ask you to arrive early in case of last-minute issues that need to be resolved, problems or questions with your laboratory studies or any other minor complications. Some waiting or downtime is an inevitable part of the process, and it is far better to expect it, be patient and have your book or iPod to pass the time. Plan to wait a little to register or check in as a patient, to have your IV started, to talk to the nurses, to talk to the doctors and to be wheeled into surgery.

Typically your lab studies will have been drawn several days or a week before your operation. Now the anesthesiologist, surgeon and operating room team will have one last look at your health and documentation, the History and Physical provided by the surgeon's office, and the preoperative x-ray (usually a chest x-ray), EKG and blood work.

If anything was profoundly abnormal in the lab work it likely will have been picked up before the day of your surgery, and your surgeon will have discussed it with you. Occasionally, however, something is missed until the day of surgery, so you have to plan for contingencies.

Every once in a while the anesthesiologist or surgeon or hospital staff realizes that for some reason the surgery has to be postponed. It doesn't happen often, but it does happen. Don't be shocked. Just roll with the punches and do whatever additional testing is required, and hopefully the situation will be resolved, and the operation can either go ahead or be rescheduled. But most of the time, even last-minute issues can be resolved. In such cases, the patient has simply spent a little more time enjoying music or a book and talking with loved ones.

This is the morning you'll meet the nursing staff. You'll change out of whatever comfortable clothes you wore to the facility and into the hospital gown countless television shows have made fun of (for good reason; you may want to ask for two gowns – one that closes in back and one that closes in front, so you don't have embarrassing exposure). Hospital or center staff will place your IV so you can receive fluids. If you do have diabetes, the nurses will check your blood sugar to make sure you're in a safe range for your operation.

At this point you'll meet the surgical team members. If I'm your surgeon, I'll come and visit with you and your support person. Our anesthesiologist will also come and spend a few minutes describing the anesthesia planned. This is the time to ask any last-minute questions or talk over any last-minute concerns and make sure I know where to find your loved ones so that I can go and talk with them as soon as the surgery is over.

And, now, it's time. You've done good, hard work preparing for your operation. You've done a great job with your exercise program, followed your liquid meal-replacement program, learned everything you can about weight-loss surgery, attended support groups and preoperative classes, worked on understanding the range of tools you'll need for success, and, most importantly, you've decided to take 100 percent responsibility for your weight loss. You're taking a very important step for your long-term health, your longevity and your quality of life, and so you're going into the operation with the most positive outlook and the most positive thoughts you can possibly have!

With that, I wish you the very best of luck.

To learn more about what exactly you need to do to succeed after surgery, I invite you to read my upcoming book on the topic of achieving long-term success after weight-loss surgery. You can pre-order a copy by visiting *www.SasseGuide.com*.

Food for Thought

» Before a weight-loss operation, you will likely have consultations with not only the surgeon but, most likely, a psychologist, nutritionist or dietician and possibly a physical trainer. You'll have the opportunity to attend support groups. Each step is an opportunity to learn and prepare for weight-loss success. Learn all you can.

» Books are a great way to get answers to questions you didn't think of when talking to your surgeon, or those questions that occur to you only in the middle of the night. See the reading guide in Appendix C.

» Audio programs are another great way to learn about successful weight loss while driving to work or working out. Visit *www.AudioDiets.com*.

» Support groups offer a way to meet other people who have already experienced the procedure you're about to undergo and ask questions from those who have experienced the operation from the inside out.

» Preoperative classes can give you the long-term tools to make your weight-loss surgical procedure a success. At Western Bariatric Institute, we offer some classes online so patients can check out teaching modules based on the specific operations they've chosen.

» In the last several weeks before your procedure you will probably be on a liquid (meal-replacement shake) diet in order to lose weight before the operation. Losing weight before the operation has a number of benefits, including shrinking the liver (which makes the procedures safer.)

» The last several weeks before your procedure will also involve an exercise program. The healthier you are going into the operation, the faster the recovery time.

» The weeks before your procedure are also time to double-check all arrangements the surgical center is making with your insurance carrier, and your own arrangements for childcare and/or eldercare during your recovery, and to double-check on your own support team.

» One week before your procedure you'll be doing the last of the blood work and medical testing.

» Two days before your procedure, double-check all arrangements – where you're supposed to be and when. The day of the surgery is a bad time to be rushed and panicky or to wind up at the wrong facility.

» The day of your procedure you do not eat. Your surgeon will advise you which prescription medicines to take. There will probably be last minute medical tests run before your procedure starts, so come prepared for short waits.

» While you may have butterflies about the operation, remember everything you've learned and how far you've come and start looking forward to your new life!

Appendix A

Western Bariatric Institute Graphs and Statistics

WESTERN BARIATRIC INSTITUTE began in 2000, and its bariatric program is a division of Western Surgical Group, the largest surgical practice in Northern Nevada. Western Bariatric Institute is a leader in the field of bariatric surgery and has a long track record of professional care, compassionate service and outstanding outcomes. Four surgeons, John Ganser, M.D., Mark Kozar, M.D., Kent Sasse, M.D., and Robert Watson, M.D., perform the surgical procedures and supervise the care of all patients. Our physicians are all experienced Board Certified surgeons, are Fellows with the American College of Surgeons and have been accredited as Center-of-Excellence physicians through the American Society for Bariatric Surgery.

At Western Bariatric Institute, my colleagues and I have performed thousands of minimally invasive laparoscopic weight-loss surgeries. The following graphs and tables illustrate some of our results over the last few years. (*See http://www.westernbariatricinstitute.com/default/About_Our_Practice for more information on our practice.*)

	LRYGB	LAGB
No. of Patients	33	176
Female/Male	32/1	145/31
Mean Age	47 (±SD 8.9, range 29-69)	46 (±SD 10.9, range 21-69)
Mean Total O.R. Time (mins)	106 (±SD 27.4, range 45-167)	75 (±SD 36.3, range 55-179)

Figure A-1: Same day surgery/outpatient surgery at two outpatient surgery centers in Northern Nevada, 2002-2007

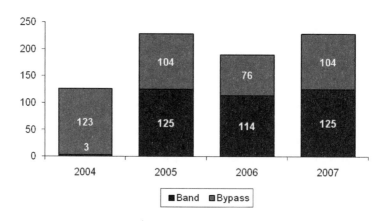

Bariatric Surgery Volume 2004-2007

Figure A-2: Number of bariatric patients at one hospital facility (not outpatient surgery), 2004-2007

LRYGB & LAGB

Follow-up (months)	Percent (%)
12	61%
9	52%
6	70%
3	82%

Figure A-3: Follow-up is very important to the success of operations. WBI works with patients after their operations. This table shows the combined percentage of follow-up at Western Bariatric Institute

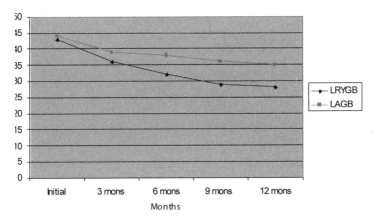

Figure A-4: Mean BMI (kg/m^2) of LRYGB and LAGB patients from initial BMI to postop 12 months.

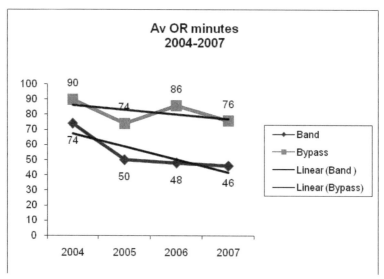

Figure A-5: Average amount of time in the OR (hospital facility)

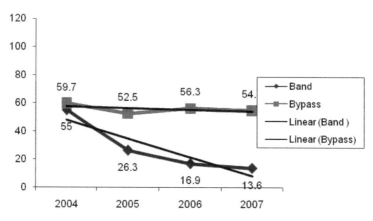

Figure A-6: How long patients spend in the hospital after their operations

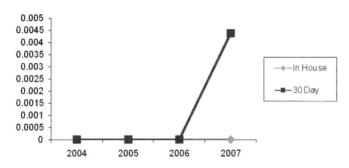

Figure A-7: Mortality rates at one hospital for LAGB and LRYGB 2004-2007 (national average was .005)

Appendix B

Recipes for Success

WESTERN BARIATRIC INSTITUTE has developed and designed a Step-by-Step meal plan to help WBI patients achieve the recommended weight loss prior to surgery and to help ease them into their liquid diets. Many people ask why pre-operative weight loss is necessary, and the simple answer is that it makes the surgical procedure safer. A 10 percent loss of excess body weight is healthier for surgery.

The meal plan below includes the liquid diet. The purpose of the liquid diet is to reduce the size of the liver, reduce abdominal fat and make the surgery safer. If the patient's body mass index (BMI) is greater than 50, the patient may need to follow the liquid diet phase of this plan for more than four weeks as directed by a surgeon at WBI.

Pre-operative Meal Plan at Western Bariatric Institute

	Step 1 Meal Plan	Step 2 Meal Plan	Step 3 Meal Plan
Breakfast	2 scoops IMetabolic protein powder with 8 fluid ounces of water	2 scoops IMetabolic protein powder with 8 fluid ounces of water	2 scoops IMetabolic protein powder with 8 fluid ounces of water
Snack	See snack list	See snack list	1 scoop IMetabolic protein powder with 4 fluid ounces of water
Lunch	Meal replacement entrée (<300 calories) and 1-2 cups of veggies (see veggies list)	2 scoops IMetabolic protein powder with 8 fluid ounces of water and 1-2 cups of veggies (see veggie list)	2 scoops IMetabolic protein powder with 8 fluid ounces of water and 1-2 cups of veggies (see veggie list)
Snack	See snack list	See snack list	1 scoop IMetabolic protein powder with 4 fluid ounces of water
Dinner	Meal replacement entrée (<300 calories) and 1-2 cups of veggies (see veggies list)	Meal replacement entrée (<300 calories) and 1-2 cups of veggies (see veggies list)	2 scoops IMetabolic protein powder with 8 fluid ounces of water and 1-2 cups of veggies (see veggie list)
Snack	1 scoop IMetabolic protein powder with 4 fluid ounces of water	2 scoops IMetabolic protein powder with 8 fluid ounces of water	2 scoops IMetabolic protein powder with 8 fluid ounces of water

Step 1

»   Can be started at any point but at least a minimum of four weeks before surgery or a minimum of six weeks before surgery if BMI is greater than 50.

»   Can be followed for several weeks but a minimum of one week

Step 2

»   Begin a minimum of three weeks prior to surgery or a minimum of five weeks prior to surgery if BMI is greater than 50

»   Follow Step 2 for a minimum of one week

Step 3

» The liquid phase

» Begin Step three a minimum of two weeks prior to surgery or a minimum of four weeks prior to surgery if BMI is greater 50 (unless directed by the bariatric surgeon)

Step-by-Step Meal Plan Vegetables List

• Asparagus	• Crookneck/Zucchini Squash
• Bean Sprouts	• Green Beans
• Bok Choy	• Green, Red, Yellow or Orange Sweet Peppers
• Broccoli	• Lettuce (up to 4 cups/day)
• Cabbage	• Mushrooms
• Carrots	• Onion
• Cauliflower	• Radishes
• Celery	• Spinach (if raw, up to 4 cups/day)
• Cucumbers	

Step-by-Step Meal Plan Snack List

FRUITS	2 Cups Honeydew Melon Cubes
1 Medium Apple, Fresh	2 Cups Watermelon Cubes
1 Medium Nectarine, Fresh	½ Small Cantaloupe
1 Medium Orange, Fresh	**DAIRY**
1 Medium Peach, Fresh	1 Piece String Cheese
1 Medium Pear, Fresh	6 Ounces Light Yogurt
1 Small Banana, Fresh	½ Cup 1% Cottage Cheese
1 Cup Blackberries, Fresh	**ADDITIONAL SNACK OPTIONS (Limit 2 Servings/Day)**
1 Cup Blueberries, Fresh	1 Cup Sugar Free Gelatin
1 Cup Raspberries, Fresh	Sugar Free Popsicle
1 Cup Strawberries, Fresh	6 Fluid Ounces V8/Tomato Juice

Amazing Shake Recipes

In the pages of Chef Dave Fouts' *Shakin' It Up* cookbook, you'll find an amazing collection of delicious shake recipes for the 21st century. For everyone who is utilizing medically recommended shakes as liquid meal-replacement, the recipes in this book serve as a wonderful resource. For who among us can truly enjoy the same "French Vanilla" flavored shake over and over again? Variety is the spice of life.

The evidence from the medical literature is clear: Meal-replacement shakes serve an important and highly effective role in weight-loss programs, whether those programs are medically-based, pre-operation or postoperation. A properly selected shake contains the protein and nutrients necessary in order to lose weight in a healthy way while controlling appetite. And now with these wonderful recipes from a chef who has had a weight-loss operation, you don't have to sacrifice flavor and variety to stick with the meal-replacement shakes and go the distance with your diet.

What Chef Dave Fouts has accomplished in the pages of *Shakin' It Up* is a sublime service – adding flavor, variety and fun to the hard work of achieving a weight-loss goal is a magical feeling. Enjoy every one of these recipes, and may they bring you even greater success on your weight-loss journey.

To order the entire collection of 20 gourmet shake recipes in Chef Dave Fouts' *Shakin' It Up* cookbook ($6.95), visit *www. iMetabolic.com* and go to the books section.

If you'd like to try any of the iMetabolic products, use code AUDIET to get a 10 percent discount off your first purchase from *www.store.imetabolic.com.*

Here are just a few of the wonderful recipes from Chef Dave:

Banana Orange Creamsicle

Banana with a splash of orange, blended to creamy perfection.
Serving size: 1

» 2 scoops vanilla-flavored protein powder
» 1 cup ice
» 4 ounces cold water
» ¼ teaspoon sugar-free orange gelatin powder
» ¼ teaspoon vanilla extract

Place cold water into blender. Add protein powder, sugar-free orange gelatin powder and vanilla extract. Blend 15-20 seconds. Add ice and blend for 30-45 seconds. Serve chilled.

Chocoholic

Double the chocolate.

Serving size: 1

- » 2   scoops chocolate flavored protein powder
- » 1   cup ice
- » 4   ounces cold water
- » 1   teaspoon sugar-free chocolate syrup
- » ¼ teaspoon butter extract

Place cold water into blender. Add protein powder, sugar-free chocolate syrup and butter extract. Blend for 15-20 seconds. Add ice and blend for 30-45 seconds. Serve chilled.

Mocha Frappaccino

Sugar-free chocolate syrup mixed with decaf coffee, blended until rich and creamy.

Serving size: 1

- » 2 scoops chocolate flavored protein powder
- » 1 cup ice
- » 4 ounces cold water
- » 1 teaspoon sugar-free chocolate syrup
- » ¼ teaspoon decaffeinated instant coffee

Place cold water into blender. Add protein powder, sugar-free chocolate syrup and instant decaf coffee. Blend for 15-20 seconds. Add ice and blend for 30-45 seconds. Serve chilled.

Appendix C

Which Band is Right for You?

With two medical device companies now each offering a laparoscopic adjustable gastric band, which band should you choose?

Up until now there has been only one laparoscopic adjustable gastric band available in the United States, the LAP-BAND®. The LAP-BAND®, now sold by Allergan, Inc., was developed by the Inamed Corporation, an American company based in Southern California. After many years of testing, and large clinical trials outside the U.S., the LAP-BAND® came to America in 2000, where its popularity has grown immensely as an effective, minimally-invasive outpatient weight-loss surgical option.

For many years, a rival band known as the "Swedish adjustable gastric band" has been in use in other parts of the world, especially Europe. The Swedish band was acquired by Johnson & Johnson Services, Inc., and its surgical instrument division, Ethicon, Inc. In 2007, the Ethicon band was granted approval for sale in the United States, so now you have a choice.

The Ethicon band has since been named the REALIZE™ Band. The REALIZE™ Band is now competing head-to-head with the LAP-BAND® after a six-year head start in the United States by Allergan's product. This new competition has lead to many questions among our patients:

» **Is there a difference between the two bands?**

» **Is one better than the other?**

» **Will surgeons offer both bands or just one?**

Like other experienced U.S. bariatric surgeons, I have extensive experience with the LAP-BAND® but less with the more recently approved REALIZE™ Band. I am well-versed on the published literature of the two medical products, and I am not a paid consultant by either company. (I discuss these subjects in even more detail in a Special Report available at *www.SasseGuide.com.*)

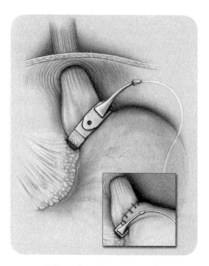

Figure d-1: The LAP-BAND®

What are the differences between these bands, and are they significant? To begin with, both bands share a great many features in common:

» Both are meant to be wrapped around the upper part of the stomach in what is essentially the identical position.

» Both have an interior balloon that lies in direct contact with the stomach, and it can be filled with saline.

» Both have tubing that connects to an access port that is placed in the deep subcutaneous abdominal wall tissue at the level of the muscles or fascia.

» Both bands act as "restrictive" procedures that lead to weight loss by restricting the stomach pouch and creating fullness and satiety.

» Both bands have more than 15 years of high-quality data supporting them and demonstrating effectiveness in weight loss and resulting health improvement.

And so both bands are remarkably similar in their design and in the way they work.

However, the REALIZE™ Band uses a slightly different design in the internal balloon. The REALIZE™ has one size and one size only. It has had very little change in its basic design for 15 years. The balloon is considered a lower pressure balloon and one that accommodates a volume of up to 10 cc of saline. Some authors believe that the REALIZE™ Band may have a lower tendency to erode into stomach tissues as a result of the low-pressure balloon, something that is a rare occurrence with either band.

The LAP-BAND® by Allergan has undergone several design changes and currently is offered in two different sizes: the "AP Standard" size and the "AP Large" size. Some surgeons find that with very large patients, and especially large men with more fatty tissue around the upper stomach, the AP Large band is easier to place and more effective. Over the years, the Allergan LAP-BAND® has gradually evolved to a large balloon size that accommodates more volume, in the range of 10 to 14 cc of saline. Both bands involve an internal balloon system that is in contact all around the stomach, where it is placed. With prior designs of the LAP-BAND®, the balloon did not reach all the way around, and this appeared to be related to a somewhat higher rate of erosion.

Another feature that distinguishes the REALIZE™ Band is a new access port that involves a mechanism to secure the port to the abdominal fascial and muscle tissue with some self-applying titanium hooks instead of hand-sewn stitches. Ethicon believes that this system will allow an easier placement of the port and will be favored by surgeons because of its convenience. Some surgeons believe this system also leads to less discomfort at the port site for the patient, an uncommon complaint in either band.

In my opinion, the currently available designs of both the REALIZE™ and the LAP-BAND® offer many very similar features, namely the circumferential 360-degree balloon and a very low risk of serious complications of erosion or slippage. Time will tell whether there are any important differences in outcomes, weight-loss results or the risk of complications over time. I believe that both of these bands share so much in common that there is unlikely to be a major difference on any of these important measures in the future.

What is clear is that each company is going to market its band with great energy and effectiveness. It is very likely that direct consumer marketing will lead to patients requesting a specific band by name. It is also likely that individual surgeons will prefer one band over another because of differences in pricing

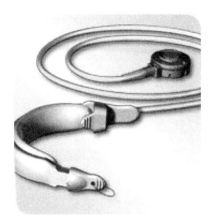

Figure D-2: The REALIZE™ Band

or ease of placement or historical familiarity. It is also the case, as with any instrument or device in the medical industry, that hospitals and surgery centers will face intense pressure to utilize only one brand of band. This pressure occurs because the manufacturers exert enormous pressures on hospitals and hospital systems to remain loyal to an entire line of products, devices and surgical instruments, or face steep price increases.

What is the Future of the Bands?

What will the future hold? With many years of high-quality studies demonstrating effective long-term weight loss and health improvements with both of these bands, it is highly likely that both of these bands will remain in the marketplace for many years to come. Now that these weight-loss medical devices are in the hands of two major medical instrument suppliers, it is also very likely that we will see increased marketing and competition.

Perhaps most importantly, increased marketing will undoubtedly spread the message about the safety and efficacy of gastric banding to more overweight people who could benefit from it. For this reason alone, tens of thousands of lives will likely be saved or prolonged in this country every year. Greater competition may also bring reduced costs for these devices down the road but may also bring more pressure on hospitals and surgery centers to align themselves with one supplier or another.

Should You Choose One Band Over the Other?

Ultimately, you should make informed choices about every aspect of your health and medical care. If you are considering the laparoscopic adjustable gastric band, then odds are that you have researched the most effective, and least invasive, ways to lose weight for the long term. In my view, a strong case can be made that either the REALIZE™ or the LAP-BAND® is a smart choice to improve long-term health, quality of life and longevity. Both appear very durable and effective for the long term, and both are placed comfortably in an outpatient setting, thus minimizing time off from work or activities. In time, factors may emerge which distinguish the bands to a greater degree, but I would recommend you talk over the topic with your surgeon and move forward when you feel comfortable with the choice you are making.

From the perspective of the health care system, the move to outpatient weight-loss surgical procedures that require less than an hour of anesthesia yet produce such profound long-term health benefits is nothing short of revolutionary. The emergence of another FDA-approved medical weight-loss device is another step in this process.

Appendix D

The Top Misadventures with Outpatient Weight-Loss Surgery and How to Avoid Them

1. A Leak

AN ANASTOMOTIC LEAK is a leak or disruption of the connection that is made in laparoscopic Roux-en-Y gastric bypass surgery between the tissues of the stomach and the small intestine. Leaks are a serious problem because they lead to a dangerous intra-abdominal infection known as peritonitis. This usually mandates a return to surgery, usually within hours of detection of the problem, to repair the leak. Sometimes this urgent complication requires an open procedure with a long midline abdominal incision. If unrecognized or not treated early, a leak can lead to serious illness, difficulty breathing and the need for prolonged intensive care unit support and care, as well as more surgery. But in the vast majority of cases, a leak will be corrected and the patient will recover with no long-term problems.

A leak, like any other complication, is best avoided entirely. If it occurs (and there is always a small percentage chance of a complication occurring), then it is best recognized very early and treated aggressively. While there is no 100 percent foolproof method of averting leaks, studies have shown that the incidence of this serious problem drops dramatically as the surgeon becomes more experienced. You can maximize your odds of avoiding this serious complication by choosing an experienced surgeon with an excellent track record. Surgeons who have managed to reduce the incidence of leaks down to the 1- or 2-percent range have done so through careful technique, avoidance of tension on the tissues and application of a regular and routine test for minor leaks either during or directly after surgery.

The signs that a leak may have occurred are high fevers, racing heart rate, increase of pain, shortness of breath, nausea and vomiting. Often all these things occur at once immediately.

The best thing you can do to prevent leaks or mitigate their effects is to put yourself in the hands of an excellent, experienced surgeon.

I have heard it suggested that overly vigorous exercise, coughing or a major fall could cause enough trauma to disrupt the suture line and create a leak, but this data is doubtful. The overwhelming majority of leaks that occur in this and any other intestinal surgery occur without any such particular trauma.

If a leak does occur you can help the surgical staff. If your nurses and surgeons are concerned about a leak, do everything you can to cooperate with investigations or studies that they want to order so that an answer can be arrived at immediately. Often the fastest and best way to both diagnose and treat a leak is to go back to surgery and operate either laparoscopically or sometimes with an open procedure.

2. Vomiting and Dehydration

Inevitably, after a person has undergone a gastrointestinal operation of any kind, the stomach and intestines will have some recovering to do before they begin working normally again. One of the most common side effects after an abdominal or gastrointestinal operation is nausea and vomiting. Anesthetic gases and pain medicines also have the side effect of causing nausea and vomiting. In most cases these symptoms appearing after a weight-loss operation do not present a very serious problem. The symptoms can be treated with anti-nausea medicines. Sometimes over the course of a few hours the symptoms can resolve and a person may still be discharged home in a timely manner without a prolonged hospital stay.

However, in a few cases, the symptoms do not subside and a person may experience persistent nausea and vomiting that requires intravenous fluids and hospitalization. The worst problem arises when these symptoms have occurred after the patient is discharged home.

What can you do about this problem? The first thing is to make sure that you are able to tolerate liquids fairly reliably before you go home. It is true that sometimes in the hustle and bustle of modern hospitals and surgery centers both patients and hospital staff are anxious to move along in the process and get the patient home in an expeditious fashion. Sometimes patients are exhibiting more optimism than realism and think that "I will be fine" even though they have not been able to hold down even two sips of sugar-free apple juice.

So, take stock of your situation and make sure that you are in fact able to drink at least a small amount over the course of a couple of hours before you make the journey home. This will give you peace of mind and avoid anxiety that stems from finding that you are not able to tolerate any oral intake.

There are a couple of other things that you can do to preempt this problem. One of them is to make sure you are very well hydrated the day and evening prior to your operation. I advise my patients to drink a good deal of extra liquids the night before an operation. This helps avoid the dehydration that can occur after an operation.

Finally, I would say that if you are at home and the nausea and vomiting occur despite your best efforts, try to intervene early with the use of anti-nausea medications. Your doctor can prescribe them (I prescribe them preoperatively so that the patient can have them on-hand, just in case), and if you use them early they may help reduce the nausea and allow you to tolerate some liquids. If the problem is persistent and doesn't look like it's going to resolve, then it is usually best to call your doctor's office. You may need to return to your doctor's office or surgical center for IV fluids. Usually after going home it is safe to wait overnight before moving to the step of returning to the hospital, but you and your doctor or the doctor's nursing staff can help advise you in that matter.

3. Heart, Lung, Kidney and Other Organ Problems

Every kind of health problem that could occur in the outside world walking down the street can occur in the hospital or in the time frame immediately following surgery. Surgery and anesthesia can both put some stress on the heart, lungs and other organ systems and can lead to some underlying problems with these organs manifesting in a serious way. Such problems are not com-

mon, but a small chance always exists of these types of issues arising. For example, people with underlying heart disease may experience heart attacks or abnormal cardiac rhythms after operations.
Likewise someone with intrinsic lung disease (for example a long-
time smoker) could experience problems breathing or develop a
lung infection. There are unlimited numbers of problems that can
occur, although complications are rare in a high-quality, high-volume bariatric surgical practice.

What can you do to protect yourself? Again, the answer is prevention. It is critically important that you notify your doctor and
your doctor's team of the underlying health problems that you
have experienced in the past. It is important not to minimize these
problems, and it is important to follow through with any recommended tests or evaluations so that these issues can be thoroughly
looked into prior to surgery and anesthesia. For example, if you
have had some heart trouble that you were told was not terribly
severe in the past, it is still important to mention it to your doctor. The doctor may want to have you undergo a cardiac stress test
just to be sure. Comply with these important investigations. They
could save you from serious postoperative complications.

4. You Think Something is Wrong, but You Can't Get Any Answers

This is an extremely frustrating problem that stems from a lack of communication from the hospital nursing staff or the surgeon and the surgeon's staff to you and your family. Sometimes there actually is no serious problem or complication but only a worry or anxiety about one. Sometimes there is a complication that is unfolding and studies are in progress to help reveal the problem, but no answers have been received. Worse, there is a serious problem and the doctor is aware of it but is too busy to communicate with you or your family.

How can you avoid this problem? The best answer lies in prevention or avoidance of the problem. As you interview surgeons and examine surgical practices, ask the questions from the beginning about communication. Ask: How will I be able to reach you, and how will you communicate with me? If I feel something is going wrong and call your office, will a nurse relay information to you and get back to me in a timely fashion? These are all reasonable questions to ask your surgeon and the surgical staff. Likewise, you can expect the outpatient surgery center staff to be in communication with you and your family if any problems or questions arise. Ninety-nine times out of 100, the surgeon, surgical staff and the outpatient surgery center staff are working hard to make your experience a positive one and are appropriately investigating potential problems or questions that arise. If a problem is ongoing, such as a reaction to medication or a potential surgical complication, generally you need to take a deep breath and give the professionals a bit of time to gain an understanding of the potential problem. So, don't expect constant and immediate communication on every issue that crosses your mind but do expect forthright communication if it appears there is a problem.

If you find yourself in the worst possible scenario, in which a serious problem is developing and no one will tell you anything about it, you need to have your allies and advocates get on the phone and call the physician's office as well as the outpatient surgery center or hospital nursing staff. Sometimes just getting an answer such as "we are getting an X-ray to check on that potential problem" is all it takes to allay anxiety.

5. Blood Clots

Blood clots in the large veins of the leg (deep vein thrombosis) used to be a fairly frequent and severe complication of weight-loss operations many years ago. This problem can cause painful leg swelling but also a potentially very serious breathing problem if a blood clot travels up the venous system to the lungs. Blood clots are more apt to occur if a person is seriously overweight, and they are more likely to occur if a person is undergoing a long operation during which time the person remains immobilized on an operating table. The blood in the venous system pools, stagnates and becomes still, like a river that stops flowing. At that point a person can develop a clot. The good news is that with modern laparoscopic weight-loss surgery, the incidence of blood clots has plummeted. In our series of approximately 3,000 cases there has been no documented blood clot occurrence.

The reason for this is probably the high level of vigilance that experienced bariatric surgeons bring to this particular problem. Most centers employ sequential compression stockings that use a pneumatic squeezing mechanism to keep the venous blood circulating in the legs. In addition, many surgeons and their staffs will also use injections of low-dose blood thinners to keep the blood from clotting abnormally.

What can you do to prevent a clot? First, ask the surgeon and the nurses about their protocol for prevention of blood clots. It would be very unusual for an experienced, high-volume weight-loss surgical center to fail to employ a vigorous blood clot prevention program.

You can also ask the surgeon how long procedures generally take. Since minimally invasive weight-loss surgery in the hands of experienced surgeons generally takes around an hour or sometimes substantially less, there is little time for blood clots to form in the legs. If your surgeon answers that routine weight-loss surgical procedures take six or seven hours, it's time to look for a different surgeon.

If after your operation you suspect that you have developed a blood clot (symptoms are a hot, red, tender, swollen calf), you need to tell your nurses and doctor immediately. A blood clot can be diagnosed with a simple ultrasound test and treated with blood thinners.

There are steps you can take to prevent blood clots from forming after surgery when you are at home resting. Be active. Move your legs. Pump your feet. Stand up and walk. Get outside. All of these recommendations are meant to keep the blood circulating and keep problems from developing.

6. Bleeding

Surgical bleeding is not as common as many people imagine, yet it is still possible for serious bleeding to occur and for a person to require blood transfusions. This kind of problem would be exceedingly rare in an LAGB procedure in an experienced surgeon's hands (probably on the order of one in 1,000 cases) and quite uncommon also in a laparoscopic RYGB procedure (in the 1-percent range). Bleeding can occur because there are blood vessels that need to be divided. There are also structures, such as the liver and spleen, that can bleed just from mild trauma to them. This can occur even with routine surgery. Bleeding is best dealt with by early recognition and treatment with either blood transfusions or a return trip to the operating room to identify and stop the source of the bleeding.

There are actually a few things you can do before your operation to reduce your risk of complications from bleeding. Your surgeon will generally advise you prior to surgery to stop taking any medicines that thin the blood and increase your chances of bleeding. These include aspirin, ibuprofen and all of the nonsteroidal anti-inflammatory type medicines. Usually it is recommended to stop these medicines five to seven days prior to an operation. In addition, if a patient is taking a more potent blood thinner called Coumadin, then the surgeon will generally advise stopping this medicine also. Special arrangements can be made for people who must have their blood thinned due to a mechanical heart valve or other special situations. Talk with your surgeon about these conditions and how to manage them.

The second thing you can do pertains to bleeding that occurs from a specific site: the liver. The liver is the largest organ in the abdomen and a place where a great deal of fat storage occurs when people gain weight. Virtually everybody who is considering a weight-loss operation has an excessive amount of fat stored in the liver, a condition which is aptly named "fatty liver" or hepatic steatosis. I describe this condition because it leads to a greater chance of fracture or bleeding from the liver during an operation, and it can be dramatically improved over the course of a mere few weeks time preoperatively.

How can you improve such a condition? By decreasing the fat storage. To accomplish this, many surgical programs ask patients to embark upon a vigorous weight-reduction and fat-reduction program lasting anywhere from two to 12 weeks before operations. This strict program consists of a liquid diet that normally runs about 800 calories per day. Several studies have shown that the liver shrinks dramatically with this preop liquid diet program, and the risk of bleeding (as well as other problems such as conversion to an open incision) are lessened with this preoperative liquid weight-loss program. So, ask your surgeon about a preoperative liquid diet. Follow the guidelines religiously. Don't cheat, and you will significantly reduce your odds of several serious problems and complications, including bleeding.

7. Conversion to an Open Operation

For many years, all weight-loss surgery was done with an open technique. This meant that a long incision was made, usually from the lower breast bone area down well below the navel. There are even a few surgeons who still argue today that this is a preferred technique even though a great deal of data and experience exists that such open surgery brings with it much longer recovery times and higher rate of complications related to the incision and wound itself. Open surgery also compromises the mechanics of the lungs and leads to greater respiratory insufficiency and respiratory complications after surgery when compared to laparoscopic surgery. With all due respect to surgeons who would still defend the open technique, it is, in my view, an antiquated technique that has been replaced by a procedure that is safer, faster and more effective: laparoscopic or minimally invasive surgery.

So what happens if your experienced laparoscopic surgeon runs into trouble and the problem can't be solved laparoscopically? The surgeon will have to convert to an open operation. This occurs in up to 2 percent of cases, even in the experienced hands of a laparoscopic surgeon performing gastric bypass surgery. It is far from the end of the world, but it would be nice to avoid this particular event since it inevitably leads to a hospital stay of at least several days, and often a week, and it brings with

it the issues related to wounds and breathing and other risks I
describe above.

Like any surgical risk, the risk of conversion to open surgery cannot be entirely avoided. However, your odds can be
improved substantially by two major preoperative efforts. One
is selecting the finest laparoscopic bariatric surgeon you possibly can, and the second is making yourself the best possible surgical candidate you can. The former involves careful research
and interviews. The latter involves working hard night and day
to improve your physical health and reduce your weight.

So, if your surgeon requires a four-week preoperative weight-
loss program, you should consider that the bare minimum.
Make a target for your own personal plan of success maximiza-
tion to lose a minimum of 30, 40, 50 or even 100 pounds prior
to your operation. This means starting a daily exercise program,
wearing a pedometer, fighting against carbohydrates, hunger
and junk food night and day, and then transitioning to a very
strict all-liquid low-calorie weight-loss program. Nearly anyone
reading this book has lost many pounds before and can do it
again; and this is perhaps the most important time in your life
for you to lose weight: prior to bariatric surgery.

It may seem a strange irony that you are seeking help to lose
weight through surgical intervention only to now be told that

in order to safely undergo surgical intervention, you must first lose weight. And yet the facts are that your risks during an operation will be significantly reduced if you lose weight beforehand. You have the power to lose pounds before your operation. For this one short-term, finite and highly important time period, you must dig deep to find the motivation and resources to lose these pounds prior to your operation. You will dramatically improve your chance of success and reduce your risk of complications, including the complication of converting to open surgery.

8. Stomach Ulcer Formation

It is increasingly recognized that stomach ulcers can form in the early weeks and months following LRYGB. This has not been found to be a significant issue with LAGB. For patients undergoing gastric bypass, however, ulcers can be a serious problem. They can lead to pain, nausea and vomiting and can become difficult to treat, sometimes causing swelling or scarring that narrows the stomach outlet, or they can result in a perforation that requires surgery. This problem has been increasingly recognized and may occur in up to 5 percent of cases after gastric bypass.

In order to avoid this, avoid agents that cause damage or irritation to the stomach lining and promote ulcers. These include, chiefly, alcohol, tobacco, nonsteroidal anti-inflammatory drugs (ibuprofen, naprosyn, etc.) and corticosteroids such as prednisone.

There may be more that you can do. It is increasingly recognized that a common bacterium known as helicobacter pylori plays a role in the formation of stomach ulcers in LRYGB as well as in the general population. So, more and more practices are now testing for the presence of this bacterium even before surgery and treating it with the antibiotics that kill it in order to lessen the chances of later stomach ulcer formation. Ask your doctor if this is a test the surgical practice performs. These measures may not completely eliminate your risk of ulcers, but the studies would suggest they would probably reduce the risks by as much as 90 percent.

9. Stomal Stenosis

There are a few different ways in which the stomach or intestines can become blocked or obstructed after LRYGB. These blockages tend to occur after someone has gone home from the hospital. The first way is that the anastomotic site of the stomach to the intestine (the connection where the stomach and intestinal limb are sewn together) scars down tightly over a few weeks. This blockage results in a gradual intolerance of foods as the person is attempting to progress to a more solid diet in the weeks follow-ing surgery. It is best treated with an endoscopy, where a lighted flexible camera is inserted down the esophagus, and the opening is gently stretched. The treatment is usually highly successful, especially if done quickly after the onset of the problem.

There is probably fairly little you can do about this preopera-tively, other than (once again) seeking a skilled and experienced laparoscopic surgeon and optimizing your preoperative weight loss, both of which make the procedure technically easier. There is evidence that the factors that lead to stenosis often involve ten-sion from the tissues, and this may be improved in part by a very successful preoperative weight-loss program. Following an opera-tion, it is important to monitor your symptoms and assess how well you are doing as you progress from liquids onward through pureed foods and on to solids. If over the course of several weeks you find that your ability to swallow and eat is worsening rather than improving, then you need to let your doctor know right away. A stenosis could be forming, and the best diagnostic test is an upper endoscopy. Long delay in recognition of the problem usually makes it much more difficult to treat and fix.

10. Constipation

Okay, constipation may not seem like a really serious problem, but it can be. One of the main reasons people become constipated after an operation is that the narcotic painkillers prescribed all cause some degree of constipation through a slowing of the bowels. Add to this the fact that you are not eating much, and it can become a bit confusing when one should expect a bowel movement. In rare cases, people may become very seriously bloated and experience pain due to constipation, which can be avoided.

Simple advice for avoiding this complication is to drink plenty of fluids in the days preceding your operation. If you have a tendency to become constipated anyway, you need to anticipate that this will likely become worse after an operation, especially if you're taking narcotic pain medication. (The most common narcotics used after bariatric operations are oxycodone, hydrocodone, codeine, morphine and hydromorphone, with trade names like Lortab, Vicodin, Norco, Percocet, Roxicet and Dilaudid.) Ask your surgeon or your nurse about this preoperatively. Take stool softeners and fiber regularly prior to the operation.

After your operation, you should expect your bowels to begin working again within three or four days. Any longer than this usually warrants treatment with a laxative.

Recovery and Beyond

Making a decision to undergo weight-loss surgery is a big step toward better health and a better life. The day you undergo the operations is the day you start a new journey. You're bound to have questions:

» **What is important?**

» **What do I eat?**

» **How do I cope with the cravings from my old life?**

» **How do I deal with people who knew me as the "fat person" I no longer am?**

» **And most importantly: What are the proven keys to weight-loss success for the long term for someone who has undergone a weight-loss operation?**

Over the years, so many people have asked me these questions that I began writing down the answers. The result is a guidebook for people who have undergone weight-loss operations and now want to maximize their success and live the fullest life possible.

The bottom line is that you can succeed in losing the weight and keeping it off forever after a weight-loss operation. All you need are the right tools. My upcoming comprehensive guide, *After Weight Loss Surgery* will give you these tools. Visit our website *www.SasseGuide.com* for this book and others in The Sasse Guide Series that will assist those on this journey.

Successful weight loss for a lifetime ...

Glossary

Anastamosis: tissue connection of the stomach pouch to the intestine

Anastamotic stricture: narrowing of the tissue connecting the stomach pouch to the intestine

ASC: Ambulatory surgery center or outpatient surgery center

Bariatric: The branch of medicine dealing with weight loss

BMI: Body Mass Index, a measure of the height and weight. Normal BMI is 18-25

Bowel obstruction: a blockage of the intestines

Cardiac arrhythmia: irregular heartbeat

CAT scan: an imaging study used for diagnostic purposes, using X-ray technology to create a 3-D image

Center of Excellence: a designation from the American Society of Metabolic and Bariatric Surgery or the American College of Surgeons denoting an experienced program that has passed certain criteria including a site inspection and satisfactory outcomes reporting

Comorbid: a coexisting illness or condition (for example, hypertension is a comorbid condition related to obesity)

Cholecystectomy: gall bladder removal

CT scan: same as CAT scan

Degenerative joint disease: wear and tear on the joints, causing arthritis and damage to cartilage and bone, often caused by and exacerbated by weight gain

Dumping syndrome: a syndrome noted by symptoms of flushing palpitation, sweating, and nausea that comes from rapid intake of sugar or high osmolality nutrients (like sugars) following gastric bypass

Endoscopy: a nonsurgical procedure to examine an organ using a flexible fiber optic tube passed down the esophagus

FDA: Food and Drug Administration

Gastric bypass: laparoscopic Roux-en-Y gastric bypass, the most popular weight-loss operation in the United States

Gastric pouch: term used to describe the small stomach pouch created in gastric bypass surgery

Gastroesophageal reflux disease: a common condition, worse with weight gain and obesity, in which stomach acid travels upward to the esophagus, usually giving an unpleasant sensation of heartburn

Gastrointestinal: pertaining to the stomach or intestinal system, digestive system

Gastrojejunal anastamosis: the area of connection from the stomach pouch to the intestine

Glycemic index: a numerical system that measures the rise in circulating blood sugar a carbohydrate triggers

Glycemic load: a ranking system for the carbohydrate content of foods based on their glycemic index and size of portions

Hypoxia: low levels of oxygen in the blood

Inferior vena cava: the large veins that bring the returning blood from the legs back to the heart

Jejunal limb: the portion of the intestine used to connect to the stomach pouch in laparoscopic Roux-en-Y gastric bypass surgery (also called Roux limb)

Keyhole incision: a small incision made on the skin of the abdominal wall in laparoscopic surgery, usually measuring 5 mm to 12 mm in length (less than half an inch)

LAGB: laparoscopic adjustable gastric band

Laparoscopic: surgery performed using a camera system and small, thin, specially designed instruments inserted through the abdominal wall, a type of minimally-invasive abdominal surgery

Laparoscopic sleeve gastrectomy: a newer weight-loss procedure in which a large portion of the stomach is removed and the remaining stomach is made into a smaller, thinner, tubular structure

LAP-BAND: the brand name of the Allergan laparoscopic adjustable gastric band

Leak: a complication of weight-loss surgery in which stomach or intestinal juice may pass outside of the stomach or intestine, causing infection or peritonitis

LRYGB: laparoscopic Roux-en-Y gastric bypass

Marginal ulcer: formation of an ulcer or sore on the inside lining of the stomach pouch

Medically supervised weight-loss program: nonsurgical physician-supervised program to lose weight, often involving diet, counseling, behavior modification and, sometimes, specially designed meals and prescription drugs

Medicare-certified: approved by Medicare, the federal national health insurance plan for the elderly and disabled

Natural orifice transluminal endoscopic surgery (NOTES): an emerging type of surgical procedure in which a natural orifice, such as the mouth, can be used to insert the surgical instruments and camera, minimizing any external incisions

Outpatient surgery: surgery in which the patient is expected to go home the same day. Often, in the eyes of insurance plans or regulators, this means within 24 hours

Outpatient surgery center (also known as **ambulatory surgery center**): a center or facility devoted to ambulatory or "day" surgery, in which patients go home after surgery, usually within 23 hours

Outpatient weight-loss operation: any of the weight-loss surgical procedures performed on an outpatient basis, in which the patient undergoes the operation and goes home within 23 hours

PCOS: polycystic ovarian syndrome, a condition involving hormonal abnormalities, weight gain and ovarian cysts

Peritoneal cavity: the space inside the abdomen where the intestines are

Pseudotumor cerebri: a brain condition that causes severe headaches

Pulmonary: having to do with the lungs

Pulmonary hypertension: an advanced state of high blood pressure in which the heart and lungs have become damaged over time

Radiology: the field of medical imaging using X-rays, ultrasound, CT scans and other imaging techniques

REALIZE™ Personal Banding Solution: the name for the Ethicon laparoscopic adjustable gastric band

Roux limb: the part of the intestine used to connect to the stomach pouch in gastric bypass surgery (also called the jejunal limb)

Satiety: the sense of feeling full or satisfied

Sleep apnea: a condition in which proper sleeping is impaired because of the floppy tissues in the throat and neck obstructing the air flow. It can range from minor snoring to severe life-threatening cessation of breathing during sleep

StomaphyX™: a new endoscopic device for revising stretched gastric pouches. It consists of a soft flexible scope passed down the esophagus with surgical instruments attached to approximate tissue and shrink the pouch. It appears promising for revision surgery.

Urinary incontinence: loss of control of the urinary bladder, resulting in involuntary passage of urine, often with coughing or sneezing

Venous stasis disease: slow transit of the blood returning from the legs upward toward the heart, resulting in swelling of the veins and soft tissues of the legs, related to obesity

Resources

Books

Weight Loss Surgery for Dummies by Marina S. Kurian, Barbara Thompson and Brian K. Davidson (For Dummies, 2005). This guide is a well-written summary of many important considerations for someone undergoing a weight-loss operation. It includes perspectives from a surgeon, a psychologist and a patient. The diagrams and explanations are clear, and the issues discussed are relevant. It has recipes, interesting subsections and points to remember, as with all the Dummies guides. It offers a balanced and accurate view of the pros and cons of most types of surgery. While the fast-changing technology has made some sections outdated, this remains a helpful resource for anyone planning to undergo weight-loss surgery.

LAP-BAND® for Life by Ariel Ortiz Lagardere (LM Publishers, 2005) offers insightful commentary from a surgeon knowledgeable about the LAP-BAND®. He covers many aspects of the process and offers one bariatric surgeon's perspective and advice on steps for patients to take.

Laparoscopic Adjustable Gastric Banding: Achieving Permanent Weight Loss with Minimally Invasive Surgery by Jessie H. Ahroni (iUniverse, 2004). This book describes the fundamental aspects of the adjustable gastric band and offers some coaching for patients.

Bariatric Support: Crossing Over to a New You by Janice Williamson and Hobart Williamson (J. Reynolds Publishing, 2005) offers nice insights for patients undergoing weight-loss operations.

The Success Habits of Weight-Loss Surgery Patients by Colleen Cook (Bariatric Support Centers Int, 2003) is a wonderful description of the habits that have proved successful for weight-loss operation patients. Ms. Cook is a patient who has researched this topic well, and she presents well-organized keys for patients undergoing weight-loss operations. She remains devoted to the field, her information is current, and she trains many support leaders throughout the country.

Weight-Loss Surgery: Finding the Thin Person Hiding Inside You, Third Edition, by Barbara Thompson (Word Association Publishers; 3rd edition, 2003) is also written by a successful gastric bypass patient who offers insightful details about her own personal journey and many helpful hints about the experience. Many readers find the information specific and valuable, told from the point of view of one who has "been there."

Ditch Your Diet in 30 Days: 90 Easy, Healthy Meal and Snack Recipes for Effective Weight Loss by Chef Dave Fouts (360 Publishing, 2009)is a terrific book of recipes from the world's first bariatric chef. Chef Dave is a successful gastric bypass patient and professional chef who turned his talents to creating healthy, safe and delicious meals for patients who have undergone weight-loss surgery. A must for any patient undergoing a weight-loss operation.

Shakin It Up by Chef Dave Fouts (360 publishing, 2008). This small book is filled with great recipes for weight-loss shakes. It makes the experience of undergoing a preoperative liquid meal-replacement diet actually enjoyable and interesting. The recipes are delicious, analyzed for calorie and nutritional value and fun to make.

Web Resources

Obesity Related Sites

Obesity Action Coalition (OAC): As a grassroots organization, OAC endeavors to bring together the individuals impacted by the life-changing disease of obesity. The OAC offers educational and advocacy information.

» *www.obesityaction.org/home/index.php*

The Obesity Society: The Obesity Society promotes research, education and advocacy to better understand, prevent and treat obesity and improve the lives of those affected

» *www.obesity.org/*

Obesity Prevention Foundation: The Obesity Prevention Foundation was established to provide communities with leadership and educational resources to combat the epidemic of childhood obesity.

» *www.obesitypreventionfoundation.org/*

National and Government Resources

CDC Division of Nutrition and Physical Activity: This Web site provides information regarding nutrition, physical activity, excessive weight and obesity, campaigns and programs, publications, recommendations, data and statistics, and training and tools.

» *www.cdc.gov/nccdphp/dnpa/*

National Heart, Lung and Blood Institute: NHLBI of the National Institutes of Health launched the Obesity Education Initiative in January 1991. The overall purpose of the initiative is to help reduce the prevalence of excessive weight along with the prevalence of physical inactivity in order to reduce the risk of coronary heart disease and overall morbidity and mortality from CHD.

» *www.nhlbi.nih.gov/*

National Institutes of Health: The official Web site of the National Institutes of Health. NIH is one of the world's foremost medical research centers.

» *www.obesityresearch.nih.gov/*

National Heart, Lung and Blood Institute: NHLBI Home Page. This site contains information for professionals and the general public about heart and vascular diseases, lung diseases and blood diseases.

» *www.nhlbi.nih.gov/*

National Institute of Arthritis and Musculoskeletal and Skin Diseases: NIAMS offers roundtable Discussion on research career paths in rheumatic diseases and Molecular Pathway in Muscle.

» *www.niams.nih.gov/*

American Heart Association: The American Heart Association is a nonprofit organization that fosters appropriate cardiac care in an effort to reduce disability and deaths caused by cardiovascular disease and stroke.

» *www.americanheart.org/presenter.jhtml?identifier=1200000*

American Cancer Society: The American Cancer Society is dedicated to eliminating cancer as a major health problem by preventing cancer, saving lives and diminishing suffering.

» *www.cancer.org/docroot/home/index.asp*

National Cancer Institute: NCI offers accurate, up-to-date, comprehensive cancer information from the U.S. government's principal agency for cancer research.

» *www.cancer.gov/*

American Dietetic Association: The American Dietetic Association is the world's largest organization of food and nutrition professionals and ADA is committed to improving the nation's health and advancing the profession of dietetics through research, education and advocacy.

» *www.eatright.org/cps/rde/xchg/ada/hs.xsl/index.html*

American Diabetes Association: The American Diabetes Association's mission is to prevent and cure diabetes and to improve the lives of all people affected by diabetes.

» *www.diabetes.org/home.jsp*

National Institute of Diabetes and Digestive and Kidney Diseases: This organization conducts and supports research on kidney, urologic, hematologic, digestive, metabolic and endocrine diseases, as well as on diabetes and nutrition.

» *www2.niddk.nih.gov/*

Bariatric Surgery

MedlinePlus: Weight Loss Surgery: a site describing research and clinical programs related to obesity.

» *www.nlm.nih.gov/medlineplus/weightlosssurgery.html*

WebMD: a general medical site with a section on weight-loss surgery.

» *www.webmd.com/diet/weight-loss-surgery/gastric-bypass*

Weight-Loss Surgery: a resource about weight-loss surgery from Allergan.

» *www.weightlosssurgeryoptions.com/*

WIN - Bariatric Surgery for Severe Obesity: government publication on obesity.

» *win.niddk.nih.gov/publications/gastric.htm*

WeightLossSurgeryCoach.com: information, inspiration and support for obese people wanting a longer, healthier life through weight-loss surgery:

» *www.weightlosssurgerycoach.com/index.shtml*

The American Society for Metabolic and Bariatric Surgery (ASMBS): the professional society for weght-loss surgeons

» *www.asbs.org/*

Obesity Help: helpful and complete information about weight-loss surgery:

>> *www.obesityhelp.com/*

WLS Lifestyles: a national publication and media outlet dedicated to providing inspiration, education and support for people struggling with obesity or maintaining a healthy weight:

>> *www.wlslifestyles.com/*

Bariatric Edge: a site maintained by Ethicon Endo-Surgery.

>> *www.bariatricedge.com/*

Gastric Bypass Information: straight answers for people seriously considering gastric bypass surgery:

>> *www.gastric-bypass-info.us/*

International Metabolic Institute: a comprehensive weight loss site offering resources for medically supervised weight-loss programs, techniques and tools, online weight-loss programs, nutritional supplements, BMI calculator, vitamins, protein shakes, diet plans and more.

>> *www.imetabolic.com/*

Sasse Guide: Dr. Sasse's personal Web site, with articles, books, information, resources and Dr. Sasse's blog all designed to be the best source of weight-loss information on the web.

>> *www.sasseguide.com/*

Western Bariatric Institute: the site for our surgical weight-loss practice

» *www.westernbariatricinstitute.com/default*

Revision weight-loss surgery: a site describing methods of revising prior weight-loss surgical procedures.

» *www.revisionweightloss.com/*

Concierge weight-loss surgery: offers a program of concentrated evaluation, counseling and coaching for patients wishing to arrange a professional destination experience for their weight-loss surgery.

» *www.conciergeweightloss.com/home*

Bariatric Surgery Articles

Gastric Bypass Surgery Articles:

» *www.locateadoc.com/articles.cfm/1454*

Sasse Guide articles and special reports

» *www.sasseguide.com/index.html#special*

Gastric Banding Surgery Articles:

» *www.locateadoc.com/articles.cfm/1454*

Mayo Clinic: bariatric surgery what can you expect:

>> *www.mayoclinic.com/health/gastric-bypass/HQ01465*

Long-term mortality after gastric bypass surgery:

>> *www.content.nejm.org/cgi/content/short/357/8/753*

Laparoscopic gastric banding: a minimally invasive surgical treatment for morbid obesity: prospective study of 500 consecutive patients:

>> *www.pubmedcentral.nih.gov/picrender.fcgi?artid=1513972&blobtype=pdf*

Audio Programs

www.audiodiets.com

Preparing for Weight Loss Surgery: An audio program outlining the essential steps to take in preparing for weight-loss surgery, beginning now and up to the morning of surgery.

An Overview of Weight-Loss Surgery: Covers all the types of weight-loss surgery and the pros and cons, risks and alternatives of each in a candid discussion from a national expert. If you are considering weight-loss surgery, then the program is a great place to start.

Diabetes and Your Future: An in-depth discussion of Diabetes, Pre-diabetes, and how to prevent it and treat it. This program focuses on the exciting recent data of successful treatment and prevention of diabetes with weight loss.

After Weight Loss Surgery: An essential how-to manual for successful weight loss after bariatric surgery.

State-of-the-Art Medical Weight Loss: An in-depth audio program discussion of what is currently the best scientifically-based medical weight-loss program available. Focuses on the data showing weight-loss success with non-surgical, medically-supervised programs and how you can take advantage of those principles for your own personal weight loss.

Vitamins and Weight Loss Surgery: This audio program covers the important topic of vitamins and vitamin deficiencies after weight-loss surgery. It outlines what the common vitamin deficiencies are before and after surgery, and how to prevent any nutritional imbalances after surgery.

Types of Weight Loss Surgery: This audio program focuses on the individual details of the different types of weight-loss surgery you may read about or hear about, from an expert surgeon who has performed them all.

Notes

1   Fleisher, L.A., Pasternak, L.R., Herbert, R., Anderson, G.F. Inpatient hospital admission and death after outpatient surgery in elderly patients: importance of patient and system characteristics and location of care. Arch Surg. 2004 Jan;139(1):67-72

2   Karlsson. J., Taft, C., Rydén, A., Sjöström, L., Sullivan, M. Ten-year trends in health-related quality of life after surgical and conventional treatment for severe obesity: the SOS intervention study. Int J Obes (Lond). 2007 Aug;31(8):1248-61. Epub 2007 Mar 13

3   Mathus-Vliegen, E.M., de Wit, L.T., Health-related quality of life after gastric banding. Br J Surg. 2007 Apr;94(4):457-65

4   Mathus-Vliegen, E.M., de Weerd, S., de Wit, L.T. Health-related quality-of-life in patients with morbid obesity after gastric banding for surgically induced weight loss. Surgery. 2004 May;135(5):489-97

5   Sjöström, L, Narbro, K., Sjöström C.D., Karason, K., Larsson, B., Wedel, H., Lystig, T., Sullivan, M., Bouchard, C., Carlsson, B., Bengtsson, C., Dahlgren, S., Gummesson, A., Jacobson, P., Karlsson, J., Lindroos, A.K., Lönroth, H., Näslund, I., Olbers, T., Stenlöf, K., Torgerson, J., Agren, G., Carlsson, L.M. Swedish obese subjects study. Effects of bariatric surgery on mortality in Swedish obese subjects. N Engl J Med. 2007 Aug 23;357(8):741-52

6   Adams, T.D., Gress, R.E., Smith, S.C., Halverson, R.C., Simper, S.C., Rosamond, W.D., Lamonte, M.J., Stroup, A.M., Hunt, S.C. Long-term mortality after gastric bypass surgery. N Engl J Med. 2007 Aug 23;357(8):753-61

7   O'Brien, P.E., Dixon, J.B., Brown, W., Schachter, L.M., Chapman, L., Burn, A.J., Dixon, M.E., Scheinkestel, C., Halket, C., Sutherland, L.J., Korin, A., Baquie, P. The laparoscopic adjustable gastric band (LAP-BAND): a prospective study of medium-term effects on weight, health and quality of life. Obes Surg. 2002 Oct;12(5):652-60

8   Bult, M.J., van Dalen, T., Muller, A.F. Surgical treatment of obesity. Eur J Endocrinol. 2008 Feb;158(2):135-45. Review

9   Perry, C.D., Hutter, M.M., Smith, D.B., Newhouse, J.P., McNeil, B.J. Survival and changes in comorbidities after bariatric surgery. Ann Surg. 2008 Jan;247(1):21-7

10   Sugerman, H.J., Wolfe, L.G., Sica, D.A., Clore, J.N. Diabetes and hypertension in severe obesity and effects of gastric bypass-induced weight loss. Ann Surg. 2003 Jun;237(6):751-6; discussion 757-8

11   Adams, T.D., Gress, R.E., Smith, S.C., Halverson, R.C., Simper, S.C., Rosamond, W.D., Lamonte, M.J., Stroup, A.M., Hunt, S.C. Long-term mortality after gastric bypass surgery. N Engl J Med. 2007 Aug 23;357(8):753-61

12   Dhabuwala, A., Cannan, R.J., Stubbs, R.S. Improvement in comorbidities following weight loss from gastric bypass surgery. Obes Surg. 2000 Oct;10(5):428-35

13   AHRQ Study Finds Weight-loss Surgeries Quadrupled in Five Years. Press Release, 2005, July 12. Agency for Healthcare Research and Quality, Rockville, MD. *http://www.ahrq.gov/news/press/pr2005/wtlosspr.htm*

14   Popularity of Weight-Loss Surgeries. Daily News Central. 2005, July 12. *http:// health.dailynewscentral.com/content/view/1265/63*

15   Powers, K., Rehrig, S., Jones, D. Financial impact of obesity and bariatric surgery. Medical Clinics of North America, Volume 91, Issue 3, Pages 321-338

16   Chohen, D. Not without its risks: Recent studies show that the incidence of bariatric surgery is growing rapidly, and that cost and safety are major concerns. 2005, Dec. *http://www.psp-interactive.com/issues/articles/2005-12_06.asp*

17   Harvard School of Public Health. Diabetes: nutrition source. *http://www.hsph.harvard.edu/nutritionsource/diabetes.html*

18   Zinzindohoue F, Chevallier JM, Douard R, Elian N, Ferraz JM, Blanche JP, Berta JL, Altman JJ, Safran D, Cugnenc PH. Laparoscopic gastric banding: a minimally invasive surgical treatment for morbid obesity: prospective study of 500 consecutive patients. Ann Surg. 2003 Jan;237(1):1-9

19   O'Brien, P.E. The LAP-ABND AP system: The platform advances. Bariatric Times. 2007. 5(5). Retrieved in Aug: *http://bariatrictimes.com/2007/06/02/the-lap-band-ap%e2%84%a2-system-the-platform-advances*

20   O'Brien, P.E., McPhail, T., Chaston, T.B., Dixon, J.B. Systematic review of medium-term weight loss after bariatric operations. Obes Surg. 2006 Aug;16(8):1032-40

21   Maggard, M.A., Shugarman, L.R., Suttorp, M., Maglione, M., Sugerman, H.J., Livingston, E.H., Nguyen, N.T., Li, Z., Mojica, W.A., Hilton, L., Rhodes, S., Morton, S.C., Shekelle, P.G. Meta-analysis: surgical treatment of obesity. Ann Intern Med. 2005 Apr 5;142(7):547-59

22   Hakala, K., Stenius-Aarniala, B., Sovijärvi, A. Effects of weight loss on peak flow variability, airways obstruction, and lung volumes in obese patients with asthma. Chest. 2000 Nov;118(5):1315-21

23 Dixon, J.B., Schachter, L.M., O'Brien, P.E.. Sleep disturbance and obesity: changes following surgically induced weight loss. Arch Intern Med. 2001 Jan 8;161(1):102-6

24 Dhabuwala, A., Cannan, R.J., Stubbs, R.S. Improvement in comorbidities following weight loss from gastric bypass surgery. Obes Surg. 2000 Oct;10(5):428-35

25 Buchwald, H., Avidor, Y., Braunwald, E., Jensen, M.D., Pories, W., Fahrbach, K., Schoelles, K.. Bariatric surgery: a systematic review and meta-analysis. JAMA. 2004 Oct 13;292(14):1724-37. Review. Erratum in: JAMA. 2005 Apr 13;293(14):1728

26 Bacci, V., Basso, M.S., Greco, F., Lamberti, R., Elmore, U., Restuccia, A., Perrotta, N., Silecchia, G., Bucci, A. Modifications of metabolic and cardiovascular risk factors after weight loss induced by laparoscopic gastric banding. Obes Surg. 2002 Feb;12(1):77-82

27 Flum DR, Dellinger EP. Impact of gastric bypass operation on survival: a population-based analysis. J Am Coll Surg. 2004 Oct;199(4):543-51

28 Pories WJ, Swanson MS, MacDonald KG, Long SB, Morris PG, Brown BM, Barakat HA, deRamon RA, Israel G, Dolezal JM, et al. Who would have thought it? An operation proves to be the most effective therapy for adult-onset diabetes mellitus. Ann Surg. 1995 Sep;222(3):339-50; discussion 350-2

29 Stratopoulos, C., Papakonstantinou, A., Terzis, I., Spiliadi, C., Dimitriades, G., Komesidou, V., Kitsanta, P., Argyrakos, T., Hadjiyannakis, E. Changes in liver histology accompanying massive weight loss after gastroplasty for morbid obesity. Obes Surg. 2005 Sep;15(8):1154-60

30 Furuya, C.K., Jr, de Oliveira, C.P., de Mello, E.S., Faintuch, J., Raskovski, A., Matsuda, M., Vezozzo, D.C., Halpern, A., Garrido, A.B., Jr, Alves, V.A., Carrilho, F.J. Effects of bariatric surgery on nonalcoholic fatty liver disease: preliminary findings after two years. J Gastroenterol Hepatol. 2007 Apr;22(4):510-4

31 Luyckx, F.H., Desaive, C., Thiry, A., Dewé, W., Scheen, A.J., Gielen, J.E., Lefèbvre, P.J. Liver abnormalities in severely obese subjects: effect of drastic weight loss after gastroplasty. Int J Obes Relat Metab Disord. 1998 Mar;22(3):222-6

32 Dixon, J.B., O'Brien, P.E. Changes in comorbidities and improvements in quality of life after LAP-BAND placement. Am J Surg. 2002 Dec;184(6B):51S-54S. Review

33 Dixon, J.B., Dixon, M.E., O'Brien, P.E. Depression in association with severe obesity: changes with weight loss. Arch Intern Med. 2003 Sep 22;163(17):2058-65

34 Schok, M., Geenen, R., van Antwerpen, T., de Wit, P., Brand, N., van Ramshorst, B. Quality of life after laparoscopic adjustable gastric banding for severe obesity: postoperative and retrospective preoperative evaluations. Obes Surg. 2000 Dec;10(6):502-8

35 Weiner, R., Datz, M., Wagner, D., Bockhorn, H. Quality-of-life outcome after laparoscopic adjustable gastric banding for morbid obesity. Obes Surg. 1999 Dec;9(6):539-45

36 Christou, N.V., Sampalis, J.S., Liberman, M., Look, D., Auger, S., McLean, A.P., MacLean, L.D., Surgery decreases long-term mortality, morbidity, and health care use in morbidly obese patients. Ann Surg. 2004 Sep;240(3):416-23; discussion 423-4

37   Klem, M.L., Wing, R.R., Chang, C.C., Lang, W., McGuire, M.T., Sugerman, H.J., Hutchison, S.L., Makovich, A.L., Hill, J.O. A case-control study of successful maintenance of a substantial weight loss: individuals who lost weight through surgery versus those who lost weight through nonsurgical means. Int J Obes Relat Metab Disord. 2000 May;24(5):573-9

38   Busetto, L., Mirabelli, D., Petroni, M.L., Mazza, M., Favretti, F., Segato, G., Chiusolo, M., Merletti, F., Balzola, F., Enzi, G. Comparative long-term mortality after laparoscopic adjustable gastric banding versus nnsurgical controls. Surg Obes Relat Dis. 2007 Sep-Oct;3(5):496-502; discussion 502

39   Becker, S. Pa. Report: ASCs save medicare $464 million annually. Jan 18, 2008. Becker's ASC review retrieved on 28th March, 2008: *http://www.beckersasc. com/ambulatory-surgery-center/surgery-center-education/pa.-report-ascs-save-medicare-464-million-annually.html*

40   Helzner, J., ASCs vs hospitals:Struggling over a flawed system. Ophthalmology Management. 2004: November. http://www.ophmanagement.com/article. aspx?article=86225

41   Outpatient Departments. Healthcare Economist. Retrieved on March 28, 2008: *http://healthcare-economist.com/2008/01/07/a-study-in-quality-ambulatory-surgery-centers-vs-hospital-outpatient-departments/http://content.healthaffairs. org/cgi/content/full/22/6/68*

42   Brechner, R.J., Farris, C., Harrison, S., Tillman, K., Salive, M., Phurrough, S. A graded, evidence-based summary of evidence for bariatric surgery. Surg Obes Relat Dis. 2005 Jul-Aug;1(4):430-41. Review

43   Ebell, M.H. Predicting mortality risk in patients undergoing bariatric surgery. Am Fam Physician. 2008 Jan 15;77(2):220-1

44 Morino, M., Toppino, M., Forestieri, P., Angrisani, L., Allaix, M.E., Scopinaro, N. Mortality after bariatric surgery: analysis of 13,871 morbidly obese patients from a national registry. Ann Surg. 2007 Dec;246(6):1002-7; discussion 1007-9

45 Fernandez, A.Z., Jr, Demaria, E.J., Tichansky, D.S., Kellum, J.M., Wolfe, L.G., Meador, J., Sugerman, H.J. Multivariate analysis of risk factors for death following gastric bypass for treatment of morbid obesity. Ann Surg. 2004 May;239(5):698-702; discussion 702-3

46 Belachew, M., Belva, P.H., Desaive, C. Long-term results of laparoscopic adjustable gastric banding for the treatment of morbid obesity. Obesity surgery. 2002, Aug 29; 12(4):564-68

47 Roux-en-Y Gastric Bypass (RYGB) is another bariatric procedure endorsed by the NIH Consensus Report on surgical treatment of severe clinical obesity. *http:// www.annecollins.com/lose_weight/roux-en-y-gastric-bypass.htm*

48 Loffredo, A., Cappuccio, M., De Luca, M., de Werra, C., Galloro, G., Naddeo, M., Forestieri, P. Three years experience with the new intragastric balloon, and a preoperative test for success with restrictive surgery. Obes Surg. 2001 Jun;11(3):330-3

49 Genco, A., Bruni, T., Doldi, S.B., Forestieri, P., Marino, M., Busetto, L., Giardiello, C., Angrisani, L., Pecchioli, L., Stornelli, P., Puglisi, F., Alkilani, M., Nigri, A., Di Lorenzo, N., Furbetta, F., Cascardo, A., Cipriano, M., Lorenzo M., Basso, N. BioEnterics Intragastric Balloon: The Italian Experience with 2,515 Patients. Obes Surg. 2005 Sep;15(8):1161-4

50 Angrisani, L., Lorenzo, M., Borrelli, V., Giuffré, M., Fonderico, C., Capece, G. Is bariatric surgery necessary after intragastric balloon treatment? Obes Surg. 2006 Sep;16(9):1135-7

51 StomaphyX™ and EsophyX™ are the names of two FDA approved medical devices
and procedures from a company called EndoGastric Solutions, based in Seat-
tle. StomaphyX™ may be useful for people who have already undergone gastric weight-loss surgery and have experienced some stretching of the stomach
pouch. EsophyX™ is a related device that works to perform stomach surgery
that solves the problem of gastroesophageal reflux, even in people who have
never before had surgery.

These two natural orifice surgical procedures involve passage of an endoscope and the use of some clever technology to suture the stomach and create
small stomach pouches or valves. It appears this new technology may already
have a role today, particularly for a subset of patients who have undergone
weight-loss surgery in the past but have failed to lose adequate weight or are
regaining their weight. A specially designed instrument allows the surgeon to
create an improvement in the stomach outflow design, so that patients will feel
more satisfaction, less hunger and resume their weight loss. Thierry Thaure,
President and Chief Executive Officer of EndoGastric Solutions, believes that
the future of stomach surgery will involve replacement of many current procedures with those that can be performed through natural orifice surgery technique, "designed to emulate proven surgical principles but from the 100 percent transoral (via the mouth) approach that requires no internal or external
incisions."

52 What is the future of weight-loss surgery? None of us has a crystal ball, but it's clear that procedures for weight loss have, in the past 10 years, become much less invasive and also much more effective at achieving weight loss.

The bar has been set very high. Future innovations will have to show that they can achieve excellent weight results to compete with the LAGB, the LRYGB and the LSG – and that won't be easy. Future innovations will also have to prove that they are less invasive or at least no more invasive and no riskier than what is available now. This will also be challenging.

It's difficult to tell at this point if the NOTES procedures will one day play a major role, but at least some of the new technology available appears to be very beneficial to patients. On the other hand, it's hard understand to how some of the new NOTES procedures (removal of the gallbladder, for instance, via an internal incision in the stomach or vagina) are any safer or better than the current standard of minimally invasive, or laparoscopic, surgery. The full scope of risks has yet to be determined, and some of the procedures that involve internal incisions will incur risks of leak or infection that may be very serious, even if rare.

I do believe endoscopic technology, like StomaphyX™, will play a role as a weight-loss procedure, at least in revising stretched pouches and possibly as a primary weight-loss procedure in the future.

So, what is the future of weight-loss surgery? I put that question to Larry Fulton, formerly the national sales director for Allergan when it introduced the LAP-BAND® and who is now Senior Director of U.S. Sales with EndoGastric Solutions.

"I see the future of weight-loss surgery as treating and studying the metabolic resolution of obesity and addressing those issues with surgery. How that will be done will be with continued improvements in surgical procedures and techniques that will allow more and more people to have this type of surgery. Safety and efficacy will be the key to the decision tree for the surgeon and patient. I believe that Endoluminal Natural Orifice Surgery will play a major role in that, not just in revision surgery but as a primary procedure as the procedure and products to support this field continue to be developed and refined."

53   Favretti, F., De Luca, M., Segato, G., Busetto, L., Ceoloni, A., Magon, A., Enzi, G. Treatment of morbid obesity with the transcend implantable gastric stimulator (IGS): a prospective survey. Obes Surg. 2004 May;14(5):666-70

54   De Luca, M., Segato, G., Busetto, L., Favretti, F., Aigner, F., Weiss, H., de Gheldere, C., Gaggiotti, G., Himpens, J., Limao, J., Scheyer, M., Toppino, M., Zurmeyer, E.L., Bottani, G., Penthaler, H., Progress in implantable gastric stimulation: summary of results of the European multi-center study. Obes Surg. 2004 Sep;14 Suppl 1:S33-9

55   Cigaina, V. Long-term follow-up of gastric stimulation for obesity: the Mestre eight-year experience. Obes Surg. 2004 Sep;14 Suppl 1:S14-22

56   Brolin, R.L., Robertson, L.B., Kenler, H.A., Cody, R.P. Weight loss and dietary intake after vertical banded gastroplasty and Roux-en-Y gastric bypass. Ann Surg. 1994 Dec;220(6):782-90

57   Balsiger, B.M., Poggio, J.L., Mai, J., Kelly, K.A., Sarr, M.G. Ten and more years after vertical banded gastroplasty as primary operation for morbid obesity. J Gastrointest Surg. 2000 Nov-Dec;4(6):598-605

58   Trus, T.L., Pope, G.D., Finlayson, S.R. National trends in utilization and outcomes of bariatric surgery. Surg Endosc. 2005 May;19(5):616-20

59   Santry, H.P., Gillen, D.L., Lauderdale, D.S. Trends in bariatric surgical procedures. JAMA. 2005 Oct 19;294(15):1909-17

60 Nguyen, N.T., Paya, M., Stevens, C.M., Mavandadi, S., Zainabadi, K., Wilson, S.E. The relationship between hospital volume and outcome in bariatric surgery at academic medical centers. Ann Surg. 2004 Oct;240(4):586-93; discussion 593-4

61 Flum, D.R., Salem, L., Elrod, J.A., Dellinger, E.P., Cheadle, A., Chan, L., Early mortality among Medicare beneficiaries undergoing bariatric surgical procedures. JAMA. 2005 Oct 19;294(15):1903-8

62 Liu, J.H., Zingmond, D., Etzioni, D.A., O'Connell, J.B., Maggard, M.A., Livingston, E.H., Liu, C.D., Ko, C.Y. Characterizing the performance and outcomes of obesity surgery in California. Am Surg. 2003 Oct;69(10):823-8

63 O'Brien, P.E., Dixon, J.B. LAP-BAND: outcomes and results. J Laparoendosc Adv Surg Tech A. 2003 Aug;13(4):265-70

64 Chapman, A.E., Kiroff, G., Game, P., Foster, B., O'Brien, P., Ham, J., Maddern, G.J. Laparoscopic adjustable gastric banding in the treatment of obesity: a systematic literature review. Surgery. 2004 Mar;135(3):326-51. Review

65 Adams, K.F., Schatzkin, A., Harris, T.B., Kipnis, V., Mouw, T., Ballard-Barbash, R., Hollenbeck, A., Leitzmann, M.F. Overweight, obesity, and mortality in a large prospective cohort of persons 50 to 71 years old. N Engl J Med. 2006 Aug 24;355(8):763-78. Epub 2006 Aug 22

66 Calle, E.E., Thun, M.J., Petrelli, J.M., Rodriguez, C., Heath, C.W., Jr. Body-mass index and mortality in a prospective cohort of U.S. adults. N Engl J Med. 1999 Oct 7;341(15):1097-105

67 Damiani, G., Pinnarelli, L., Sammarco, A., Sommella, L., Francucci, M., Ricciardi, W. Postoperative pulmonary function in open versus laparoscopic cholecystectomy: A meta-analysis of the Tiffenau Index. Dig Surg. 2008 Jan 30;25(1):1-7

68 Karayiannakis, A.J., Makri, G.G., Mantzioka, A., Karousos, D., Karatzas, G. Postoperative pulmonary function after laparoscopic and open cholecystectomy. Br J Anaesth. 1996 Oct;77(4):448-52

69 Zacks, S.L., Sandler, R.S., Rutledge, R., Brown, R.S., Jr. A population-based cohort study comparing laparoscopic cholecystectomy and open cholecystectomy. Am J Gastroenterol. 2002 Feb;97(2):334-40

70 Staph infections are more common because of the impaired blood supply through the extensive subcutaneous fat. The infection-fighting and prevention cells of the body have to travel to the skin to prevent infections, and obesity make that travel more difficult.

71 Suter, M., Giusti, V., Héraief, E., Calmes, J.M. Band erosion after laparoscopic gastric banding: occurrence and results after conversion to Roux-en-Y gastric bypass. Obes Surg. 2004 Mar;14(3):381-6

72 Suter, M., Calmes, J.M., Paroz, A., Giusti, V. A 10-year experience with laparoscopic gastric banding for morbid obesity: high long-term complication and failure rates. Obes Surg. 2006 Jul;16(7):829-35

73 Weiner, R., Blanco-Engert, R., Weiner, S., Matkowitz, R., Schaefer, L., Pomhoff, I. Outcome after laparoscopic adjustable gastric banding – eight years experience. Obes Surg. 2003 Jun;13(3):427-34

74 Weiner, R.A., Weiner, S., Pomhoff, I., Jacobi, C., Makarewicz, W., Weigand, G. Laparoscopic sleeve gastrectomy – influence of sleeve size and resected gastric volume. Obes Surg. 2007 Oct;17(10):1297-305

75 Mognol, P., Chosidow, D., Marmuse, J.P. Laparoscopic sleeve gastrectomy (LSG): review of a new bariatric procedure and initial results. Surg Technol Int. 2006;15:47-52. Review

76 Cottam, D., Qureshi, F.G., Mattar, S.G., Sharma, S., Holover, S., Bonanomi, G., Ramanathan, R., Schauer, P. Laparoscopic sleeve gastrectomy as an initial weight-loss procedure for high-risk patients with morbid obesity. Surg Endosc. 2006 Jun;20(6):859-63. Epub 2006 Apr 22

77 Braghetto, I., Korn, O., Valladares, H., Gutiérrez, L., Csendes, A., Debandi, A., Castillo, J., Rodríguez, A., Burgos, A.M., Brunet, L. Laparoscopic sleeve gastrectomy: surgical technique, indications and clinical results. Obes Surg. 2007 Nov;17(11):1442-50

78 Garcia, V.F., DeMaria, E.J., Adolescent bariatric surgery: treatment delayed, treatment denied, a crisis invited. Obes Surg. 2006 Jan;16(1):1-4

79 Sugerman, H.J., Sugerman, E.L., DeMaria, E.J., Kellum, J.M., Kennedy, C., Mowery, Y., Wolfe, L.G. Bariatric surgery for severely obese adolescents. J Gastrointest Surg. 2003 Jan;7(1):102-7; discussion 107-8

80 Collins, J., Mattar, S., Qureshi, F., Warman, J., Ramanathan, R., Schauer, P., Eid, G. Initial outcomes of laparoscopic Roux-en-Y gastric bypass in morbidly obese adolescents. Surg Obes Relat Dis. 2007 Mar-Apr;3(2):147-52

81 Dillard, B.E. III, Gorodner, V., Galvani, C., Holterman, M., Browne, A., Gallo, A., Horgan, S., Le Holterman, A.X. Initial experience with the adjustable gastric band in morbidly obese U.S. adolescents and recommendations for further investigation. J Pediatr Gastroenterol Nutr. 2007 Aug;45(2):240-6

82 SUMMARY OF CLINICAL MEASURES AND DATA

    a. Measurements at baseline (one to six months before surgery) and at approximately one month, three months, six months, nine months and twelve months after surgery, and then annually thereafter:

        ii.   Weight

        iii. BMI (Body Mass Index)

      iv.   Resolution/development of comorbid conditions

  b. Height

  c. Total weight loss

  d. Percent weight loss

PARTICIPANTS

Number of Subjects: The study population will consist of 25-50 adolescent (15-18 years old) patients who are undergoing or have undergone laparoscopic adjustable gastric band operation performed by a bariatric surgeon at Western Bariatric Institute (WBI).

Inclusion Criteria: The subject may be enrolled if he/she meets all the following criteria:

a. Male or female subject 15-18 years old and is scheduled to have laparoscopic adjustable gastric band procedure.

b. The subject meets criteria for gastric bypass surgery as outlined by National Institutes for Health (NIH).

c. The subject has completed a bariatric surgery screening visit with a physician at WBI.

d. The subject has a physician's referral for a preoperative nutrition evaluation and postoperative fellow-up visit.

e. The subject is given written informed consent prior to enrolling in the study.

f. The subject has the physical, motivational, and intellectual ability to understand and follow all aspects of study requirement.

Exclusion Criteria: Subjects will be excluded from the study for any of the following reasons:

a. The subject does not meet the criteria for bariatric surgery as outlined by the National Institutes for Health.

b. The subject is not physically, motivationally and intellectually able to understand and follow all aspects of study requirement.

c. The subject is not willing to participate in both the nutrition evaluation and postoperative follow-up visit.

d. The subject has not completed a bariatric surgery screening visit with a physician at WBI.

e. The subject does not have a physician's referral for a preoperative nutrition evaluation and postoperative follow-up visit.

f. The subject is not willing to consent to release of data.

83 Busetto, L., Angrisani, L., Basso, N., Favretti, F., Furbetta, F., Lorenzo, M.; Italian Group for LAP-BAND. Safety and efficacy of laparoscopic adjustable gastric banding in the elderly. Obesity (Silver Spring). 2008 Feb;16(2):334-8

84 Taylor, C.J., Layani, L., Laparoscopic adjustable gastric banding in patients > or =60 years old: is it worthwhile? Obes Surg. 2006 Dec;16(12):1579-83

85 Sugerman, H.J., DeMaria, E.J., Kellum, J. Sugerman, E.L., Meador, J.G., Wolfe, L.G. Effects of bariatric surgery on older patients. Annals of Surgery. 240(2):243-247, August 2004

86 Papasavas, P.K., Gagné, D.J., Kelly, J., Caushaj, P.F., Laparoscopic Roux-En-Y gastric bypass is a safe and effective operation for the treatment of morbid obesity in patients older than 55 years. Obes Surg. 2004 Sep;14(8):1056-61

87 HCUP Fact Book No. 9: Ambulatory Surgery in U.S. Hospitals, 2003 (continued) Part II: Detailed Statistics for Selected Procedures and Populations Procedures Influenced by Technological Advances. Retrieved on April 30, 2008 from: *http://www.ahrq.gov/data/hcup/factbk9/factbk9c.htm*

» In 2003, only 3 percent of bariatric surgeries performed outpatient

» Mean age for bariatric operation patients 42 years, inpatient or outpatient

» Almost all bariatric surgeries performed outpatient in patients ages 18 to 64 (55.7 percent in patients ages 18 to 44 and 42.9 percent in patients ages 45 to 64)

» Nearly 83 percent of outpatient bariatric surgeries performed on females

» Private insurers billed for eight out of 10 outpatient bariatric operations. 5 percent of outpatient operations billed to government insurance programs (i.e., Medicare and Medicaid)

» Rate of outpatient bariatric surgeries billed to uninsured patients was almost 5 times rate of inpatient bariatric surgeries billed to this group (11.6 percent versus 2.4 percent). This finding may reflect surgeries among patients who are otherwise insured, but opt to self-pay for outpatient bariatric surgery, which is often less expensive, when bariatric surgery is not a covered benefit.

88 Regi Schindler of BLIS, Inc., a company currently providing such insurance or warranty coverage, puts it this way: "If everyone pays a little bit more for the premium, then very few people will have to be exposed to financial hardship should a complication arise."

89 Dávila-Cervantes, A., Domínguez-Cherit, G., Borunda, D., Gamino, R., Vargas-Vorackova, F., González-Barranco, J., Herrera, M.F. Impact of surgically-induced weight loss on respiratory function: a prospective analysis. Obes Surg. 2004 Nov-Dec;14(10):1389-92

90 Thomas, P.S., Cowen, E.R., Hulands, G., Milledge, J.S. Respiratory function in the morbidly obese before and after weight loss. Thorax. 1989 May;44(5):382-6

91 Sabar, R., Kaye, A.D., Frost, E.A., Perioperative considerations for the patient on herbal medicines. Middle East J Anesthesiol. 2001 Oct;16(3):287-314. Review

92 Kaye, A.D., Kucera, I., Sabar, R.. Perioperative anesthesia clinical considerations of alternative medicines. Anesthesiol Clin North America. 2004 Mar;22(1):125-39. Review

Index

Other books in the 'A Sasse Guide Series' by 360 Publishing available in 2009

Check *www.SasseGuide.com for availability and ordering*

E-Books Available

Weight-Loss Surgery for Adolescents

Weight-Loss Surgery for Seniors

Weight-Loss Surgery: Which One is Right For You? The Cutting Edge of Weight-Loss Surgery Information

After Weight Loss Surgery: The Keys to Weight-Loss Success After Bariatric Surgery

Doctor's Orders: 101 Medically-Proven Tips for Losing Weight

by Kent Sasse MD, MPH, FACS

This simple yet powerful tips resource provides meaningful evidence-based practical and effective tips for initial weight loss and long-term weight maintenance. It touches on key topics that help remind us to initiate and ingrain long-term healthy behaviors. It points out small meaningful steps that we can all take on the road to a healthier weight. Tips like, "Serve your meal on a smaller plate", seem simple, and yet remind ourselves that these are the steps that lead to long-term weight loss. Scientific studies demonstrate that we consume 40% less food when it is served on a smaller plate! Take advantage of Dr. Sasse's insight and reading of the scientific literature to make your own weight loss journey a success.

Ditch Your Diet in 30 Days
90 Easy, Healthy Meal and Snack Recipes for Effective Weight Loss

by Chef Dave Fouts and Vicki Bovee, M.S., R.D.

This cookbook provides a systematic meal plan for 30 days encompassing five meals per day while maintaining a 1200 calorie per day intake routine. From shopping lists to complete nutritional panels, this cookbook provides everything from A to Z that one needs to bring variety, nutritional balance, and delicious meals to not only the bariatric surgical community but also anyone that is seeking delicious meal ideas that help maintain proper nutritional balance.

Shakin' it Up

**by Chef Dave Fouts with Nutritional Consultation by
Vicki Bovee, M.S., R.D.**

This recipe book delivers wonderful and creative shake recipes from a trained chef who has undergone bariatric surgery himself and understands the need for diversity and flavor during these very important phases before and after surgery. In addition, this book is valuable to anyone making meal replacements a normal part of their weight loss and weight maintenance routines.

Smooth Foods

**by Chef Dave Fouts with Nutritional Consultation by
Vicki Bovee, M.S., R.D.**

This recipe book focuses on the second eating phase after weight loss surgery, when smooth, easy-to-digest foods are the order of the day. Having undergone weight loss surgery himself, Chef Dave Fouts provides delicious ideas from Creamy Scrambled Eggs to Crab Louie to Greek Bean Salad. All recipes are geared toward providing variety with sound nutrition while still focusing on the protein, vitamin, and texture needs of anyone who has undergone weight-loss surgery.